THE COMPLETE BOOK OF

COSMETIC

**Dennis P. Cirillo, M.D., and
Mark Rubinstein, M.D.**

FACIAL SURGERY

A Step-by-Step Guide to the Physical and Psychological Experience, by a Plastic Surgeon and a Psychiatrist

SIMON AND SCHUSTER

NEW YORK

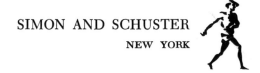

Copyright © 1984 by Dennis P. Cirillo and Mark Rubinstein
All rights reserved
including the right of reproduction
in whole or in part in any form
Published by Simon and Schuster
A Division of Simon & Schuster, Inc.
Simon & Schuster Building
Rockefeller Center
1230 Avenue of the Americas
New York, New York 10020
SIMON AND SCHUSTER and colophon are registered trademarks of
Simon & Schuster, Inc.
Designed by Eve Kirch
Manufactured in the United States of America

10   9   8   7   6   5   4   3   2   1

Library of Congress Cataloging in Publication Data
Cirillo, Dennis P.
  The complete book of cosmetic facial surgery.
  Includes index.
  1. Face—Surgery.   2. Surgery, Plastic.   I. Rubinstein,
Mark,   II. Title.
RD119.5.F33C57   1984   617'.52   84–1397
ISBN 0–671–47743–9

To Katy and Joshua

Contents

Introduction   11

Part One: Preparing for Cosmetic Facial Surgery

1. Finding the Proper Surgeon   15
2. Your Consultation   19
3. About Anesthesia and Surgery   43

Part Two: Surgical Procedures

4. Surgery of the Nose   53
5. Facial Contouring   75
6. Cosmetic Eyelid Surgery   85
7. Face-Lift Surgery   101
8. Brow and Forehead Surgery   129
9. Chemical Peeling and Dermabrasion   139
10. Collagen Treatments   149
11. Other Surgical Procedures   155
12. Looking and Feeling Great   169

Index   171

ACKNOWLEDGMENTS

We wish to express our gratitude to Dexter Cirillo and Linda Sutter for their helpful suggestions and creative input throughout every phase of this book. Vincent Juliano made the photographs possible and Susan Sheffield Smith graciously consented to model. We owe a special debt of gratitude to our editor, John Herman, who helped us conceive and write this book.

Introduction

In the last decade there has been a dramatic increase in attention to health, fitness and self-image. With so much emphasis on well-being and an attractive appearance, plastic surgery has come of age. No longer the province of the rich and famous, plastic surgery today is available to more people than ever before. Each year many thousands of people turn back the clock with cosmetic facial surgery. And the numbers are increasing!

Why would a plastic surgeon and a psychiatrist write a book about cosmetic surgery?

Over the years we have treated many patients, both separately and working together. With time, we became more aware of the many questions and concerns people have when contemplating cosmetic surgery. There are a host of questions about the surgery itself (whether it's nasal surgery, a face-lift or any other procedure); and there are anxieties and doubts about what to expect before, during and after the operation. We discovered that—more than anything else—patients want to *understand their surgery*, and that they want and need to know exactly what to expect—physically and emotionally—during the entire surgical experience.

Drawn from our experience with patients, this book was conceived as a means to answer your questions and to deal with your concerns. It provides a complete, step-by-step approach to understanding your surgery. It presents comprehensive, practical advice

11

about choosing a plastic surgeon, about anesthesia and about the various surgical procedures you may undergo. Each operation is clearly explained and demystified. The book explores the nature of your relationship with your doctor and explains what you should realistically expect to learn in your consultation with a plastic surgeon.

We have divided the book into two sections: Part One, "Preparing for Cosmetic Facial Surgery," which should be read by everyone, and Part Two, "Surgical Procedures," with individual chapters devoted to each type of operation.

We have provided clear, easy-to-understand diagrams of operations throughout. There are before-and-after photographs of patients who have undergone cosmetic surgery. There are explanations of postoperative do's and don'ts, of possible side effects and of possible complications. There are vivid, true-life case histories of patients we have treated in our practices.

Cosmetic surgery is elective—it is something you choose to do. With this choice, however, there often go many self-doubts and anxieties. In this book, and in the questions and answers following each section, we address these emotional issues. Expect to find your very own questions answered in these pages—some of them questions you would feel uncomfortable discussing with your family, your closest friends, or even with a plastic surgeon!

Facial cosmetic surgery marks a milestone in your life. It is an enormous personal decision on the road to self-improvement. This book can be your *complete* and practical guidebook, if you are contemplating or are about to have cosmetic facial surgery. We wish to provide you with practical advice on handling the *entire cosmetic surgery experience* as both a physical and an emotional event.

We hope this book will fill a special need for the hundreds of thousands of patients (and their families) who have this surgery each year. In the following pages we intend to share our professional experience with and insights into the physical and emotional dimensions of plastic surgery.

DENNIS P. CIRILLO, M.D.
MARK RUBINSTEIN, M.D.

PART ONE

PREPARING FOR COSMETIC FACIAL SURGERY

ONE

Finding the Proper Surgeon

Cosmetic facial surgery should be one of the milestones in your life, a special event that makes you look better and feel better about yourself! If you are seriously considering such surgery, the first step is to consult with a properly trained surgeon. How do you choose a surgeon who will reshape your looks for the rest of your life? This may be one of the most important decisions you will ever make. The following are some guidelines to help you find a surgeon suitable for your needs.

- A referral by a friend. Knowing someone who has had successful cosmetic surgery is important. You have the recommendation of someone you know and trust and, even more helpful, you can see an example of the surgeon's work. There is no substitute for good results! But this is only a beginning. You should meet with the doctor *yourself* so you can determine whether the surgeon can meet your specific cosmetic needs.
- A recommendation by your family physician. It is best if your physician knows a surgeon to whom he has referred patients in the past. This is certainly better than having your doctor give you a "blind" referral to a surgeon in the area. Such a blind referral may

be helpful, but you should know if your family doctor has seen the results of the surgeon's work.

• Inquiring on your own. When looking for a cosmetic surgeon, you must know what credentials he or she should possess.

To insure that practitioners have fine skills and proper training in a certain specialty, the medical profession throughout the United States has established specialty board-certification.

Board certification and specialty societies can be confusing because there are so many of them. Certain specialists besides board-certified plastic surgeons claim to be qualified to do cosmetic facial surgery. Some otolaryngologists (ear, nose and throat specialists) and certain ophthalmologists perform cosmetic facial surgery. How do you choose the best specialist for you? You *must* inquire about the surgeon's qualifications and experience. Here are some helpful tips:

Your surgeon should be a board-certified specialist who, after his or her training in general surgery, devoted a large portion of residency training to cosmetic surgery. In our view, board-certified plastic and reconstructive surgeons are most likely to satisfy this requirement.

Your surgeon should frequently perform the type of surgery you yourself are seeking. For instance, if you are interested in a face-lift, your surgeon's practice should be devoted largely to cosmetic facial surgery, rather than surgery of some other area of the body.

Here are some other ways to ensure that the surgeon you visit is properly trained and qualified.

Local hospital and county medical societies will refer you to a qualified doctor in any specialty. Such societies are listed in any local telephone directory.

You may consult the *Directory of Medical Specialists.* This volume, available in most libraries, lists all board-certified physicians by their specialties and by the areas where they practice.

If you have any questions about a plastic surgeon's qualifications you may contact the American Society of Plastic and Reconstructive Surgeons. This society is located at 233 North Michigan Avenue, Chicago, Illinois 60601, and maintains a nationwide referral service. You may telephone the society at (312) 856-1818 for a list of board-certified plastic surgeons in your area anywhere in the United States.

While you are visiting with a surgeon, the nature of the consultation should help you decide if the surgeon is the right one for you. Have a complete consultation. This means visiting the surgeon at his or her office. This crucial meeting with your prospective surgeon is so important that we have devoted the next chapter to it. A number of components go into a thorough consultation, but you must find a surgeon who will:

—Frankly discuss in detail the feature you wish to improve
—Allow you to ask questions freely
—Ask you questions about your feelings and concerns relating to your proposed surgery
—Explain the surgical procedure and postoperative regime
—Show you examples of his or her work (using preoperative and postoperative photographs of other patients)
—Discuss fees and give you an overall picture of the operation's expenses

Choose a surgeon who takes the time to explain your proposed surgery in a clear and complete way. If you feel that the doctor is too busy to spend time with you, you may have the wrong physician for your needs. You might do well to consult with someone else.

Trust your senses. Is it easy to establish a rapport with your surgeon during the consultation? Do you feel comfortable with this physician? In a consultation with a plastic surgeon, you are seeking out a skilled professional service, one about which you need to learn as much as you can. Does the surgeon answer your questions frankly? Do you feel the doctor is interested in your specific esthetic problem? Are the doctor's recommendations tailored for you, or do you feel you are just another number coming through the consultation room? Remember, you and your surgeon will be a team whose goal is to help you look as good as you can. You must be able to work well together!

If you combine all these factors, your chances of finding a qualified and experienced surgeon are excellent. Such a surgeon is a board-certified specialist doing predominantly cosmetic facial surgery; who does many such operations each year; who operated on someone you know; who comes highly recommended by other professionals; who shows you preoperative and postoperative photographs of former patients with results you find acceptable; who explains the surgery to you and with whom you feel a comfortable rapport—such a surgeon is most likely to have the skills and experience to help you achieve your desired cosmetic results.

Today, a great deal of cosmetic facial surgery is done in clinics or in the doctor's office. This is fine provided the outpatient facility has the same emergency care equipment and trained personnel available as that in a hospital setting. If your surgeon operates a clinic or does surgery in the office, ask if it is fully equipped.

Once you decide to have surgery, make certain the fee for the operation is established in advance. Find out about hospital and clinic charges. There is usually no fee for follow-up care after your surgery. Also learn which costs, if any, are covered by insurance. Do not be surprised if, after you have decided to have surgery, the surgeon's secretary requests payment for the operation in advance. This is commonly done. Cosmetic surgery, being elective, is rarely covered by health insurance plans. You are fully responsible for payment of the fee. Your surgeon will usually request payment at or before the time of your operation.

Make certain to learn about these things in advance. There should be no unpleasant surprises when you are considering facial surgery.

TWO

Your Consultation

It isn't easy to walk into a surgeon's office, especially if it is your first contact with a surgeon. Suddenly you find yourself in a waiting room, about to speak to someone you've never before met. And you are going to ask the surgeon to change a vital part of your appearance. If you aren't slightly nervous, then something is wrong. Most people thinking about cosmetic facial surgery have questions, concerns and anxieties about the consultation and the proposed operation.

Questions Patients Frequently Ask Themselves

We have found that people very often bring the following questions and concerns into the consultation room, *even before meeting with the surgeon.*

What is possible for me?

Can my nose be made smaller or more shapely? Can my eyes look less tired? Can my face be made to look as young as I feel? Most people have genuine concerns about any proposed surgery. They wonder if they can really be helped. In your consultation you should want to know about *your specific* cosmetic problem. You *should* want to know if it can be treated and if your looks can be improved. These questions are completely valid! After all, every patient consulting with a plastic surgeon feels that he or she needs some improvement. It is perfectly natural to wonder about your problem and if it can be significantly helped.

Do I really need this surgery?

Most people consulting with a plastic surgeon have doubts about cosmetic facial surgery. It is elective surgery. It is something you choose to do. It is not essential to your health. Most people view surgery as something done only for illness. It may feel strange to have a free choice in something as important as surgery. This choice may make you feel slightly anxious.

However, though you don't *need* such surgery in the strict medical sense, this does not invalidate the important decision you make to look and feel better about yourself. Many people considering cosmetic surgery have the same doubts and concerns you do. If you have a bump on your nose, or if you feel you look older than you should, then cosmetic surgery is a perfectly acceptable answer to these problems. The decision to have a consultation for cosmetic facial surgery is an important first step toward self-improvement.

This is a luxury operation. Will I feel guilty about taking up a bed?

Perhaps surprisingly, this is a common feeling people have before their consultations with a plastic surgeon. Strictly speaking, cosmetic facial surgery is not a necessity. This does not make it wrong or ill-advised. If you are a good candidate for such surgery and want to have it done, that is sufficient to make it right for you.

Rest assured that hospitals with plastic surgeons on their staffs have ample provisions for cosmetic surgery patients. You will not take up a bed ordinarily reserved for a sick patient. Traditionally, hospitals are associated in people's minds with illness and life-threatening situations. Since cosmetic surgery does not fall into such a category, over the last few years many plastic surgeons have been performing surgery in their offices or in outpatient surgical clinics. If you wish, you may arrange for surgery at such a facility.

If I don't have this surgery now, will I ever get up the courage again?

Doubtless you've come for a consultation after thinking about it for a long time—you may have considered the idea for years! Perhaps you are worried that people will think you are vain, or you may be anxious about surgery or about changing your looks. Finally, you have taken the first step—you have arranged for a consultation! Now that you have gone this far, you may feel a sense of urgency about having surgery.

However, you should take your time. Cosmetic surgery is elective —there is no need to rush into anything. Allow yourself to digest the information you will be gathering in your consultation. Your consultation is a vital process during which you will learn about your cosmetic problem and how best to deal with it. Avoid feeling as though it's a now-or-never situation. You may even wish to consult with more than one surgeon, if this helps you make a decision. Remember, a consultation does not obligate you to have surgery. Taking your time can help you find the best surgeon for your cosmetic problem.

Even though I've come for this consultation, I'm afraid of surgery.

It is difficult to imagine any prospective patient with no concerns or anxieties about a surgical procedure. The *idea* of an operation alone can be frightening. This is why your consultation with a plastic surgeon is so important.

Your consultation should be a fact-finding period when you should learn a great deal about the proposed surgery. You should learn what is possible and reasonable *for you* in view of *your specific* cosmetic problem. A free-flowing discussion with your surgeon should make you feel much more confident about any proposed surgery. The more you know about the surgery and about what to expect before and after the operation, the less frightened you will be.

I've heard that after a nose job, my nose will be weaker. Or, I've heard that a face-lift will "fall" in two years.

There are many myths about cosmetic facial surgery. You may come to your consultation with a great deal of *hearsay information* you've gathered from friends and relatives. In our experience, these bits of hearsay are usually the focus of people's anxieties during their consultations. We hope to dispel these myths as we describe each cosmetic surgical procedure later in this book.

The time you spend with your surgeon should provide you with solid facts and sound information. Only when you have learned as much as possible about the proposed surgery can you make a sensible decision about having cosmetic facial surgery.

I'm tired of looking the way I do and I finally want to do something to change my looks.

Many people feel handicapped because of their looks. They may come for a consultation with a plastic surgeon feeling they have to justify the decision to have cosmetic facial surgery. Dissatisfaction with one's nose or with the signs of aging is justification enough. A consultation is reasonable if you are truly interested in learning how your looks may be improved.

After you arrive at your consultation, you may find yourself wondering about some of the following questions: How many times has this doctor performed this kind of surgery? Does he think I'm strange to want an operation? Will he really know what I'm looking for? Can my appearance be changed the way I'd like it to be? What will I look like after an operation? Are there any dangers in this? Any complications? And what will all this cost?

These are some of the questions you may want to ask during your consultation. All your questions should be answered to your satisfaction. The consultation should not be viewed as one meeting; we prefer to think of it as a series of meetings. The number of meetings prior to any operation will vary depending upon your surgeon and the individual needs you have as a patient.

Are You Well Suited for Cosmetic Surgery?

Over the years, surgeons and psychologists have found that certain attitudes indicate that cosmetic surgery is appropriate for a patient.

Is There a Real Flaw or Imperfection?

First, is there really a cosmetic flaw that lends itself to surgical correction? Do you have a large nasal hump or a bulbous tip? Is your face sagging? Does your chin appear flawed or unharmonious with the rest of your face? Does this flaw lend itself to improvement?

Are You Motivated for Yourself?

You are better suited for cosmetic facial surgery if you wish to please *yourself*, not your family or friends.

REGINA R. came for a consultation accompanied by her mother. Regina's mother seemed more eager for the surgery than Regina did. After I questioned them further, the following facts came to light: Mrs. R. had undergone a rhinoplasty 18 years earlier, and Regina's nose was identical to her mother's former nose. It was an unpleasant reminder to Mrs. R. of her own looks prior to surgery. Regina herself had little interest in changing her nose. She had come to please her mother. I did not feel that surgery was proper at that time and recommended that Mrs. R. see Dr. Rubinstein for a consultation. She did so and accepted our recommendation that surgery not be done. Regina herself would decide how she wished to look for the rest of her life.

Can you honestly say to yourself, "I want this operation even if no one but me *ever* notices anything about me has changed?" If so, then you are a good candidate for surgery.

Are Your Goals Well Defined?

The person who, upon entering the surgeon's consultation room, asks a vague, unfocused question such as, "What can you do to make me look better? I haven't liked the way I look for years," is not a good candidate for cosmetic surgery. This person has no clear goal.

Are Your Expectations of Surgery Realistic?

Do you understand that your features may be changed for the better, but that cosmetic surgery *cannot* bring about personality changes or magical transformations of any kind? The person whose hopes and expectations of surgery are far-fetched and who sees surgery as a passport to a new life is not a good candidate for facial cosmetic surgery.

> ROGER L. was a 26-year-old man who came to me for surgical consultation. He quickly produced a glossy photograph of Paul McCartney and requested that I make him look like the former Beatle. It was clear that Roger L. was not a good candidate for surgery.

The extent of an actual imperfection may have little to do with someone's dissatisfaction with his or her face. We have seen people in our practices who, despite actually being handsome or beautiful, have long been discontented about a minor imperfection. In addition to the physical flaw, there may be an enormous psychological component to a person's view of himself or herself. For some people, the physical problem may be only the tip of an iceberg. A feature may become a symbol for *everything* someone feels is wrong in life. In such a case it makes more sense to explore how to change bad feelings rather than your face.

The First Meeting: Establishing a Rapport

The first meeting between you and your surgeon is crucial. Your entire cosmetic surgical experience is affected by the impressions formed here. The essence of the consultation is to establish *communication* between you and your physician. This first meeting allows you and your physician to gather pertinent information about each other and about your cosmetic problem.

Take advantage of your consultation. Ask all the questions you feel are important. The more you know about the doctor's professional qualifications and about the operation, the more confident you will feel. Asking questions and learning about the surgery are the essence of your role in the consultation!

Some people have trouble asking doctors questions. They often fear that they will seem ignorant or will offend the physician. You are not wasting your doctor's time by asking questions. Any physician genuinely interested in patients *will welcome* questions. Questions help the surgeon understand your problem. The surgeon needs input from *you* so your cosmetic problem can be clearly defined and treated. You must think of your physician as part of a team of which you are a member.

In this initial meeting you and your surgeon should establish a rapport. You should feel your surgeon is interested in any concerns you have. It would be impractical to list and answer all these questions now—we will do so later in the appropriate chapters. There will also be a section devoted to frequently asked questions at the end of each chapter. But if you have any concern about surgery, you should bring it up with your surgeon at the *very first meeting in your consultation!*

During the consultation, there should be a frank discussion about whatever feature you wish to improve. A surgeon doing a proper job will ask *you* certain questions. Which specific part of your feature do you wish to change? How long have you been dissatisfied? Why do you want plastic surgery *now*?

Getting on the Same Esthetic Wavelength

The surgeon should then examine your face. He will be making a medical and esthetic assessment of your cosmetic problem so that he can offer recommendations that are tailor-made for you.

Part of this consultation should include examining photographs of your face. These medical-grade photographs are usually taken by a member of the surgeon's staff or by a professional photographer. These photographs will help give you a clear picture of the intended surgery. The surgeon can demonstrate exactly where the incisions will be placed and what changes the surgery will make in your appearance. All this helps you develop reasonable and realistic goals for your surgery. Examining your photographs with a surgical expert gives you the opportunity to show the physician which areas concern you the most. Is it the tip of your nose? Or the hump in the middle? Is it the puffy bags beneath your eyes? Is it the jowls beneath your jaw? Or a sagging neckline? Using photographs, you can point out to the surgeon which changes you would like and discuss them in detail.

In communicating with your surgeon, the most important step is for both of you to establish a *common esthetic language*.

When proposing to alter your nose, for example, we must be absolutely certain of what we're talking about. The words "scoop," "bump" and "hook" (words often used by patients), or even quantitative terms such as "broad" and "narrow," are vague and may mean different things to you and to your surgeon. It is here that *photographs are imperative*, so that you are both discussing *your* features with the same mental imagery.

For this reason, preoperative photographs are indispensable. These pictures serve several purposes. First, they enable you and your surgeon to see your features objectively. Specific contours and parts of the face may be studied in as quantitative a way as possible. The relationship of these parts to each other and to the rest of your face (your facial harmony) can also be critically examined.

The photographs also serve as a working frame of reference for the surgeon in planning the operation. They can also be used for reference by the surgeon in your absence and during the operation. And after the surgery, they allow for a comparison with your pre-operative appearance.

Another useful tool to arrive at this mutual esthetic language is in the nature of a homework assignment. Here the surgeon may ask you to collect photographs of faces with features you both "love" and "hate." Magazines are an excellent source of such photos. This is not a frivolous exercise; rather, it lets you crystallize your own ideas and preferences and helps the surgeon learn more about the changes you hope to have.

Above all, this photographic review helps establish an "esthetic wavelength" between you and your surgeon. In examining the pictures, you and your physician may decide which feature(s) should be changed and how they may best be altered. We stress the point that the effort to alter looks is a *mutual* one.

One of the most unpleasant things to contemplate is having cosmetic facial surgery only to end up with a look that you dislike. A photographic review helps prevent such a painful surprise. Let's say you wish your nasal tip to be thinner and more delicate (more definition or sculpting). These words are then translated into a photograph. You then have a visual goal, and you and your surgeon may define together the meaning of such terms as "too thick" or "too thin." Skillful questioning by the surgeon allows for more specific information about the final shape you wish your features to assume. (For instance, how straight should the new profile be, or to what extent do you wish to have definition or sculpting in the area of the nasal tip?) Using photographs and questions, the surgeon may determine how realistic your expectations are.

What are the boundaries of what surgery can and cannot accomplish? Here too, photographs are helpful. Cosmetic surgery may indeed bring your features into greater balance and harmony (we will see this in photographs as we progress). If your nose has a bulbous tip, it may be made to look more natural and less conspicuous. If it has a large hump in the upper area, it may be brought into alignment with your other features. But none of this is magic and there are real limitations to the possibilities. If you have a broad face with wide features and widely set eyes and thick skin, you will not, after surgery, end up with a thin, delicate, refined nose. Even if you could, such a nose would look misplaced in conjunction with your other features. Your facial features, your skin, the underlying cartilage and bone and your healing capacity all play a part in the outcome and set limitations on the cosmetic changes you can reasonably hope for. Using photographs helps the surgeon demonstrate the limits of what can and cannot be done.

Still another tool is photographs of other patients on whom your surgeon has operated. This may help you feel more confident about your surgeon. And it adds another dimension to the consultation. By comparing results of patients with similar problems, you can arrive at a more accurate indication of the possible outcome.

During this photographic review, *your* unique esthetic wavelength emerges, and this helps bring into focus what looks good for *you*. This can make the goal of esthetic change an easier one to obtain.

As with most esthetics, there are choices. No single "look" or result is the only or best one. A skilled surgeon is as interested as you are in examining various choices and in helping you achieve the most pleasing result. The entire process should be a mutual effort by you and your physician. Together you can decide how best to change your features and resolve your esthetic problem.

Subsequent Meetings

The purpose of subsequent meetings is to gather more information, which often involves an examination of the preoperative photographs. Don't expect to be flattered by these black-and-white pictures. Their purpose is to highlight what's wrong with your features, not to send to your friends.

A free-flowing discussion about these pictures allows you to define your esthetic problem and determine how to correct it. During this process it should become clearer what can or cannot be done in surgery. You will also review the pictures you were requested to bring in. You might at this point also wish to inspect preoperative and postoperative photographs of other patients.

NORMA B. illustrates the importance of subsequent meetings. She was a 19-year-old woman who came with her parents for a consultation. She hoped that a large nasal hump could be reduced. Norma and her parents thought that her main esthetic problem was the hump. I agreed, but noted to myself that Norma's chin was markedly recessed, a feature which *by itself* would have made her nose seem protuberant. I said nothing about this at the time. At the end of this meeting I asked Norma to obtain medical-grade photographs.

At our next meeting, using photographs, I demonstrated how Norma's recessed chin was part of her esthetic problem. It was clear that a chin augmentation (in addition to the nose surgery) would result in a far more pleasing profile and in greater facial harmony. Some weeks later, after a third meeting, the rhinoplasty and chin augmentation were done. Norma and her parents were very happy with the results.

Preoperative Considerations

Your surgeon should take time to explain the preoperative procedure, including any tests which may be necessary. How long will the procedure take? Where will it be done—in the office or in a hospital? What should you expect to happen before the operation? What is the postoperative regime? What are the possible complications of this surgery? The answers to these questions vary from operation to operation; we will discuss them in each relevant chapter.

During your consultation your surgeon should also take a detailed medical history, noting any medical conditions (no matter how minor) and any medications you take on a regular basis. You should mention even the most innocuous over-the-counter medications to your physician. For instance, both vitamin E and aspirin can promote bleeding during your operation. They should be changed or discontinued, if possible, prior to surgery.

Some surgeons recommend that preoperative patients begin a special diet to help reduce swelling and promote healing. These diets vary from physician to physician and depend on the particular patient's medical needs.

Your surgeon should take the time to discuss any questions, concerns or reservations you have about surgery or anesthesia. As we said before, you should view your consultation as a series of meetings; the actual number is determined by how comfortable and informed you feel about the operation. Some people may wish to get an opinion from a second surgeon. Do not hesitate to do this if it makes you more comfortable. This is going to be *your* surgery!

It is often helpful for a spouse or family members to be present during the consultation. This is especially important if these family members will be with you during your postoperative recovery period. The presence of your family will probably make your postoperative recovery period safer and freer from anxiety.

When to Have Cosmetic Facial Surgery?

There is no absolute rule about the timing of an operation. Some surgeons do not operate on someone whose life has recently undergone a major change or trauma. You should expect your surgeon to ask about these issues. Your surgeon may want you to avoid surgery while you are dealing with another important emotional issue.

MRS. K. was a 58-year-old woman whom I saw in consultation. She wanted to change her nose, the one feature she'd been unhappy with all her life. After careful questioning it became clear that Mrs. K's husband had died six months earlier. This had wrought enormously complex emotional changes in her. In a sense, she was trying to rearrange not just her nose, but certain things in her life. While she'd always been discontented with her nose, it had now become a symbol of her sadness and discontent. If she could change this one unacceptable feature, her life, so she thought, would become more interesting and filled with bright things. Mrs. K. was dealing with her emotional turmoil by focusing on her nose. I recommended that she wait an additional twelve months before seriously considering surgery. If after having dealt more fully with the loss of her husband she still wished to have surgery, it could then be done.

Some people may unwittingly be searching in an operation for something that no surgery can possibly provide. While most people requesting plastic surgery are reasonably motivated, there are some instances where it makes more sense for the patient to explore how to change unpleasant inner feelings rather than unwanted outer features. Both Mrs. K's timing *and* her motivation for surgery were inappropriate.

You should not feel pressured to make a decision about having surgery. Your consultation is a fact-finding period. Many people have doubts and reservations during the consultation—and afterward. After all, the decision to have surgery to alter your looks is a milestone in your life. There are very few people who would entertain no doubts about such a matter.

Any reservations should be discussed with your surgeon. Your physician should willingly answer any remaining questions about the operation. This by itself is often reassuring. Again, lack of information is your enemy. After discussing your doubts and concerns with your doctor, most of them will disappear.

If any reservations persist, you should not hesitate to postpone the operation. Don't be afraid to discuss this with your doctor— your surgeon does *not* want to operate on a hesitant or reluctant patient. Some people have trouble telling this to a physician. They may feel that first wanting an operation and then deciding against it is backing down, or that they are disappointing the physician— or even being disloyal. Try to eliminate such thoughts from your mind.

Don't be surprised if, after you express such doubts, *your doctor* suggests postponing the operation until you've further explored your hesitation. Your surgeon may even recommend psychological counseling. This does not mean your physician thinks you are disturbed! It merely indicates the doctor's awareness of your concerns, which may be alleviated by talking with a professional.

DR. CIRILLO:

BARBARA L., a 26-year-old woman, came to my office requesting nose surgery. She was accompanied by her husband, who mildly objected to the operation. He said he was happy with Barbara's looks, but he agreed that if she wanted the surgery he would not object.

After the consultation, Barbara decided to have her nose reduced in size.

On the day of the operation, while her husband was driving her to the hospital, Barbara became extremely nervous. Suddenly she felt she could not go through with it. At the hospital she burst into tears, saying she wanted the surgery but was frightened. The operation was postponed and I suggested that Barbara meet with Dr. Rubinstein.

DR. RUBINSTEIN:

When the couple met with me, Barbara admitted that her husband's objections had worried her. "What if I look 'different' afterward?" she asked. Would her husband still be attracted to her? Her husband tried to reassure her, saying he had objected because he'd wanted her to know he was happy with her as she was. She did not have to change her looks to please him.

We occasionally see a patient who is afraid of changing his or her looks. Most of us feel comfortably familiar with the way we look, even if there is a feature that may not be pleasing. Some people may be fearful of changing what is familiar. We all have an image of the way we look, and changing this may seem frightening. Rest assured, however, that cosmetic facial surgery does not seek to alter one's look radically. The best results are often obtained when a subtle change is made, and when facial features become more harmonious.

Since Barbara's anxiety had begun on the way to the

hospital, I asked Barbara to tell me about any thoughts she
might have had in the car. At first she could not recall any. After
some questioning, Barbara suddenly remembered that she had
been thinking about the anesthesia. That was when she became
nervous. I asked her about anesthesia, and she was able to
recall having, as a young child, been "knocked out" prior to a
tonsillectomy. She was afraid of repeating that frightening
experience.

DR. CIRILLO:

Barbara, her husband and Dr. Rubinstein discussed anesthesia and her fears about it. Some time later, Barbara returned
to my office and the operation was done. Barbara and her
husband were both very pleased with the results.

Fees and Other Arrangements

During the consultation the surgeon should state the full
fee for the operation. Hospital and clinic fees should also be discussed. You should discuss your insurance with the surgeon and
determine if your surgery, or any part of it, will be covered. You
should also discuss after-care and follow-up treatment. Most
surgeons do not charge an additional fee for such follow-up treatment, but regard it as part of the cost of the surgery. In short, you
should know exactly what your surgery will cost before you enter
the operating suite.

If you decide to have surgery, you and your surgeon should
discuss anesthesia. We will talk about this important topic in the
next chapter.

Once you decide to have an operation, your surgeon will make
arrangements at the hospital or clinic facility where the operation
will be performed.

You should make arrangements to take sufficient time off from
work or school or home duties to allow for a restful recuperation
after the surgery. You should completely discuss this postoperative
period with your surgeon. The physician should explain how this

period of time will be spent, the precautions you must take, the approximate period of time you must refrain from strenuous activity, and so on.

You should know if there is going to be any postoperative swelling after your cosmetic facial surgery. How long will such swelling take to subside? Not knowing what to expect after your operation can lead to an unpleasant postoperative experience. We will discuss in detail in the appropriate chapters the postoperative period for each surgical procedure.

About Change

Some patients worry about reactions of friends and relatives. "What will they think when they see my new nose?" It may sound surprising, but when you've had surgery with good results, there is very little dramatic commentary from friends or relatives. Sometimes there is none. You may be amazed when someone you haven't seen in a few years does not even notice your changed looks! You are encountering the psychology of change. After noting the difference in your appearance, people usually accept the change without further thought. The new look becomes as much your image as your appearance had been prior to the change.

Some people have a specific concern about others' reactions to their new profile: "Will friends think I'm vain for having had cosmetic surgery?" Others worry about the reactions of relatives: "Will there be resentment? Will they think I'm trying to get rid of my family heritage?"

There is a valid general rule about this: If you are happy with the results, the people who care about you will be happy for you and will support you. As we mentioned before, in a short while your new look will be your regular look. Everyone will seem to forget you had surgery.

While friends and relatives may forget your old look, a very real change *has* taken place in your looks. You should be prepared for this. We treated a young woman who, after nose surgery, had to deal with real changes in her life. Simply put, she was much better looking! Before the surgery her social life had been meager, whereas she was now more popular. This change was not an automatic prescription for happiness. Rather, she found herself receiving requests for dates and felt uncomfortable with all this new-found male attention. It took her many months to adjust to her new status as an attractive woman.

About the Post-Op Blues

Occasionally a patient becomes sad or depressed after cosmetic surgery. This is rare and usually not serious. It generally happens because not enough time was taken to explain the surgery to the patient beforehand, and to explore the patient's motivations and expectations. This further emphasizes the importance of communication between the patient and the surgeon.

The key thing to remember is that surgery is a *process* requiring time and adjustment. It is not a magical bolt of lightning bringing with it immense life changes. The most effective way of preventing the post-op blues is simply knowing beforehand what to expect after surgery. You must also know the realistic limitations of what surgery can and cannot do. If you don't believe in magic, you won't be disappointed when no magic is forthcoming.

If you are suffering from the post-op blues, a frank discussion with your surgeon can often help clear the air.

DR. CIRILLO:

ALICE B. came to see me for a consultation. It was two weeks after she had had a rhinoplasty with another surgeon. She was very depressed and worried. She still had some swelling and some discoloration. During the consultation she said she was disappointed and uncertain about her new nose. Alice B. told me her surgeon had said everything would be fine and that she would be seen in six months for a follow-up. In fact, the results were acceptable. Alice did not know what to expect in her postoperative regime. With a little reassurance and in-depth explanation about the healing period, Alice felt much better.

Very rarely, a postoperative patient may become seriously de-pressed. Such feelings may linger and may not fade despite reassur-ances and the passing of time. Though this is a rare occurrence, you should know about depression. Here are the major signs:

> Loss of interest in activities which were once pleasurable.
> Change of appetite and weight loss or weight gain.
> Sad or dejected mood with crying spells. Feelings of pessi-mism and helplessness.
> Fatigue, often coupled with sleeplessness, particularly awakening early each morning and not being able to get back to sleep.

Most often, if someone becomes depressed following cosmetic surgery, the depression has nothing to do with the surgery itself, but has been triggered by the experience of the surgery. The patient may have had unrealistic expectations and is disappointed when such expectations are not fulfilled. (For instance, no surgical face-lift can make someone feel so young that he or she can come out of retirement and resume full-time work at a former position. Or, no face-lift can make up for the loss of dear friends or relatives.)

If depression occurs, it can be treated. A qualified psychiatrist should be contacted. Depending on the severity of the depression, the psychiatrist may use psychotherapy or medication along with psychotherapy. It is important to realize that if depression occurs in someone who has undergone cosmetic surgery there is a good chance the patient has been struggling with deeper emotional con-flicts all the while.

About Looking Good

If you have had a consultation with a plastic surgeon and have decided to embark on this important means of self-improvement, you have taken an enormous step in a new direction. If surgery is done properly, the results can make you feel better about your looks and yourself.

But surgery is only part of the overall project you have undertaken to look better. There are other important steps to consider if you wish to look and feel as good as you can. These steps are so important that we have chosen to enumerate them here, before we describe the specific cosmetic surgical procedures. These vital steps include:

A sensible dietary regime to control seesawing weight gains and losses. Good nutrition with the proper caloric intake is essential for your general health and well-being. This is important at all ages, but it becomes more so as we get older. One of the most damaging effects of fluctuating weight is upon the skin of the face and neck. When someone gains 15 to 20 pounds, the excess weight is distributed throughout the body. Much of it is stored in the fatty deposits beneath the skin, especially in the lower face and neck area. After losing weight, many people find that their skin does not shrink back to its former tight fit over the underlying muscles. This can cause the skin to sag and wrinkle.

A new style of makeup or a new hairdo may be an important complement to the positive changes in your face. A more suitable style to your hair or a more appropriate makeup can greatly enhance your looks. Do not be surprised if your surgeon recommends a consultation with experts in these areas for helpful tips about enhancing the benefits you derive from your cosmetic surgery.

MRS. A. was a 55-year-old woman who came to me complaining that only one year after her face-lift (which had been done by another physician) she felt she already looked much older. After an examination of her face, I asked about her dietary habits. She admitted that she had gained and lost 20 pounds twice in the year since her surgery. She had lapsed back into earlier habits of poor weight control and of ignoring her hair and makeup.

I advised her that she did not require surgery. Rather, she should maintain a sensible diet, and should consider consulting with a beauty expert.

After six months of weight control and after having her hairstyle and color changed, Mrs. A. had a much more vibrant and youthful appearance.

—Avoid excessive use of alcohol. Alcohol, in sufficient quantity, can cause general health problems and may create a puffy, swollen appearance about the eyes.

—Avoid smoking. Aside from considerations of general health, smoking affects blood vessels by making them "stiffer," a process known as atherosclerosis, or hardening of the arteries. This can add to the tendency to bleed more than usual in an operation.

—Take sensible steps to protect your facial skin from the harmful effects of the sun. The sun is an enemy to your skin. You should use total sunblocks when enjoying outdoor activities during the summer months. Although a tan may look becoming, repeated overexposure to the sun hastens aging of the skin.

Cosmetic facial surgery alone will not keep you trim, young or vibrant. It may be a start, but there is more you must do. Good dietary habits, regular sleep, not smoking, precautions with the sun, and a sensible exercise program are essentials in any serious self-improvement program. These measures, coupled with freedom from severe emotional stress, are necessary if you want to look and feel as good as you can.

Frequently Asked Questions

What does the term "plastic" in plastic surgery mean?

The word *plastic* is derived from the Greek word meaning "to shape" and has nothing to do with the modern-day synthetic material we call plastic. Plastic surgery is the surgical specialty involved with reshaping various features of the face and body.

You advise that one be realistic about surgery and its results. What exactly is realistic?

Being realistic is knowing what you can or cannot expect. Changing your nose or eliminating some other cosmetic flaw will not change *you*. It is not a magical passport to something new or wonderful. It can be a way of correcting an esthetic flaw about which you've felt uncomfortable or self-conscious. It may enable you to feel better about your looks and about yourself and may lead to a greater sense of well-being. These are the only miracles to expect.

Is plastic surgery a kind of psychotherapy?

Surgery is never psychotherapy. However, if by psychotherapy you mean something that makes you feel better, then almost anything qualifies as psychotherapy. Well-motivated and realistic patients with esthetic problems may find that, following successful surgery, they feel better about their looks and about themselves. While this is not psychotherapy, it can be a great step toward self-improvement and better feelings.

Can I come out looking worse that I did before surgery?

Since much about appearance is subjective, there is the possibility you may not like your results. The worst thing for a patient to encounter is a postoperative result that he or she dislikes. For this reason, it is very important to spend time during your consultation gathering as much information as you can about the operation and about your potential postoperative looks. This places additional importance on the preoperative photographs and on establishing an esthetic wavelength with your surgeon during the consultation. This maximizes your chances of knowing how you will look after surgery, so that you will most likely be satisfied with the results. When having facial surgery of any kind, the last thing anyone wants is to be surprised.

I've heard that some patients, after having cosmetic surgery (a nose job or a face-lift), first feel very happy, even "high." Then, they have a severe letdown. Is this true?

In our experience, most patients who are properly motivated for cosmetic facial surgery, and who have taken time to learn about their proposed surgery, are very pleased with their results. The case you mention of a patient first being very euphoric and then becoming depressed is an illustration of someone who may have had unrealistic expectations of surgery and who did not learn what to expect post-operatively.

I'm a man and I'm considering cosmetic surgery. Will I feel out of place in the surgeon's waiting room? I've heard that most cosmetic surgery patients are women.

Nowadays, more and more men are having cosmetic facial surgery. There are no precise statistics, and the percentage of men consulting with a cosmetic surgeon may vary from one physician to another. Some cosmetic surgeons report that as many as 25 percent of their patients are men.

If I see a plastic surgeon for three or four visits (a consultation) doesn't this begin to become expensive?

There is no "correct" or "proper" number of visits to have with your plastic surgeon during the consultation period. You should spend as much time as you reasonably feel *you* need to become knowledgeable about the surgery and to feel comfortable. This may occur in only one meeting or may require two, three or more sessions together. Most plastic surgeons regard the consultation as open-ended. In many instances, one fee covers a reasonable number of consultation sessions.

You say I should feel free to get another opinion if I feel this is necessary. If I consult with another surgeon (or two other surgeons) won't this become costly?

The most important aspects of your consultation are learning about your proposed surgery and feeling you have established a rapport and an esthetic "wavelength" with your surgeon. If you feel these important factors are missing you should seek another opinion. It is far better to pay for one additional consultation than to go through surgery when you feel uncertain about the operation or the surgeon.

Is it appropriate for me to bring my husband (wife) along for the initial consultation?

Yes. You should do whatever you need to do in order to feel comfortable and confident during this milestone period of your life. Your spouse will be better able to understand you and better prepared to help you during the postoperative phase. Your spouse may help you recall the surgeon's preoperative instructions. Your spouse's presence at your consultation will enrich his or her understanding of your experience, will help foster realistic expectations for both of you, and can be a meaningful shared experience.

THREE

About Anesthesia and Surgery

The Preoperative Procedure

You have completed a consultation with a plastic surgeon and have decided to have cosmetic facial surgery. Once a date is set, you must prepare for the operation. Preoperative instructions vary from one surgical procedure to another, and we will discuss them specifically in each appropriate chapter. Here, however, are some general preoperative considerations.

Before any surgery is done, you must have a complete physical examination. This should include x-rays and laboratory tests. This examination may be at your family physician's office or at the facility you are entering for your surgery. This examination should be shortly before the surgery, to ensure that you are in good health for the operation.

You should take nothing by mouth after midnight the night before surgery, and you should not eat breakfast that morning. This is so that your stomach remains empty, lessening the likelihood of any interference with your anesthesia.

On the morning of your surgery, you will check into the facility where the operation will be done. You will meet the surgical and nursing staff who will assist in the operation and will be taking care of you.

Before the operation, an intravenous catheter will be placed in your arm so that medication may be quickly and painlessly administered during surgery. In the rest of this chapter ("About Anesthesia") we·will explain all you need to know about this important part of your experience so you will be relaxed and anxiety-free during your surgery.

About Anesthesia

Whichever cosmetic surgical procedure you have, it will require anesthesia. It is important to know as much as possible about anesthesia, so that you feel confident your surgery will be painless and anxiety-free.

Most people have heard the terms "general" and "local" anesthesia. With general anesthesia the patient is put to sleep. This anesthesia is usually associated with "serious" operations. Many people have experienced local anesthesia in the dentist's chair. Here, a specific area of the body is numbed by the local injection of medication at the site where the procedure will be performed.

Today, with the great advances in anesthesia, an entire spectrum exists between local and general anesthesia to eliminate pain and to minimize anxiety. Here is how it works.

Before the operation either a nurse-anesthetist, working under the direction of the surgeon, or an anesthesiologist visits the patient. This medical specialist should take sufficient time to meet the patient and evaluate the patient's concerns or anxieties about the operation and anesthesia. Then a thin intravenous catheter is inserted into a vein in the arm. This open pipeline is imperative during *any* surgery. Should the patient require additional medication for any reason, such medication can be given quickly and safely through the catheter.

Before placement of the catheter, a sedative or tranquilizer (Valium, for example) may be given orally. This induces a pleasant state of drowsiness. Additional sedation may be given by mouth or through the intravenous catheter. This allows the local anesthetic (given in the operating room) to be injected without any unpleasant sensations.

The local anesthesia is then injected into the area where the operation will take place, along with a small amount of adrenalin, which causes the small blood vessels of the area to constrict. This helps to minimize bleeding, while the anesthetic "blocks" or "freezes" the tissues so no pain is felt.

The drowsiness induced by the intravenous sedative may become a twilight sleep. Some patients experience a sense of well-being bordering on euphoria. Others may feel completely unconscious, even though, medically speaking, they are only lightly anesthetized. They can respond to commands and even answer questions. When performing cosmetic surgery on the face, most surgeons prefer this state to total unconsciousness because the operation is done on a face that is not completely relaxed. (The muscles of a deeply anesthetized patient's face are so relaxed that they lose their usual tone.) The patient's wakefulness also allows the surgeon to give commands (look up; look down; open your mouth; show me your teeth; raise your eyebrows), and the amount of excess tissue to be removed is more easily estimated.

Another advantage of sedation is that medications may be used to block out all memory of the operation. The patient recalls either a pleasant twilight state or remembers nothing. The patient is comfortably relaxed during the operation. Breathing, heartbeat and other vital functions remain strong and steady the entire time.

Some patients prefer being put to sleep. They want their surgery in a state of complete oblivion, wishing to wake up without any memory of the operation. Others prefer being fully aware of everything in the operating room. They want to retain a sense of control over mind and body, wishing to recall the surgery clearly and completely. These patients may request minimal sedation—enough for relaxation—but not enough to cause drowsiness.

As many people know from visits to the dentist, a pain-free procedure does not guarantee that there will be no anxiety. Some find lying or sitting back (in a dental chair or an operating room) very trying, even though it is painless. *There is no need to endure anxiety during an operation!* It is important to know that the combination of anesthetics can alleviate this. By regulating the amount of sedative given, the patient can be made to feel comfortably anxiety-free while surgery proceeds painlessly.

Another option may be medical hypnosis for pain and anxiety control. This is not at present a popular method of anesthesia, but evidence is accumulating to indicate that hypnosis may become more widely used for cosmetic surgery in the future.

Possible Aftereffects of Anesthesia

There may be some aftereffects of anesthesia.

Some people have a slight feeling of nausea during the immediate postoperative period. This will pass quickly.

Some people may vomit, but this is infrequent.

Some patients may feel slightly lethargic for the first few hours after surgery. This will wear off.

These possible consequences of anesthesia are not necessarily dose-related. Rather, they depend on how you individually react to the anesthesia. Some people may have aftereffects even with slight amounts of sedation. These minor problems make it mandatory that you be observed during the immediate postoperative period. A trained nursing staff must be available, and should you experience any unpleasant feelings after surgery, do not hesitate to call on these professionals.

We have outlined the basics you need to know about anesthesia for cosmetic facial surgery. Most important to remember is that anesthesia is an integral part of your surgical experience. You should know as much about it as possible. Not knowing enough invites feelings of helplessness and anxiety. These unpleasant feelings are needless. You should thoroughly discuss anesthesia with your surgeon *before* you enter the hospital or clinic for your cosmetic surgery.

Frequently Asked Questions

I am frightened of any altered state of consciousness. Is this normal?

Yes, this is normal. Most people are reluctant to be put to sleep, or to have partial unconsciousness induced, by medication or hypnosis. Some people may feel they are losing control, which makes them nervous. There is no irreversible change or alteration in your consciousness. There is usually a pleasant drowsiness (depending on the amount of medication given) followed by some mildly euphoric feelings or by a state of restful sleep. When the operation is over you are completely awake. Any mild drowsiness will disappear in a short while and you will be your normal self.

If I have surgery with sedation, for how long afterward will I remain drowsy?

This varies according to how much sedation is given during the surgery. Some people are more sensitive to medication and may stay sleepy longer. Most patients find that after an hour or two they are no longer tired. There are new medications available that allow the surgeon quickly to reverse the soporific effects of the sedative without waiting for it to wear off.

What happens if during surgery I get nervous? I don't want to be frightened at such a time.

During surgery the physician can easily monitor a patient's emotional state. If a patient gets nervous, edgy or agitated, more sedative or tranquilizer can be given through the intravenous catheter. This is painless and very quick. Within moments the patient feels calmer and may even fall asleep. There is no need to feel tense or anxious during surgery.

Are there risks associated with anesthesia?

There are risks associated with anesthesia, with any operation (no matter how seemingly simple), and with every medication (even with aspirin). No surgical intervention in the body's normal workings is totally risk-free. However, cosmetic surgery, done properly by skilled professionals in the proper facility, has minimal associated risks. There are very few complications associated with anesthesia when used with a healthy patient.

I'm more nervous about anesthesia than about surgery. Is this normal?

This is often the case. Many people have anticipatory anxiety about anesthesia, although they feel confident about the surgery. You should learn as much as you need to know about the kind of anesthesia that will work best for *you*. You and your surgeon can plan your anesthesia together, specifically to meet your individual needs and preferences. Your surgeon should be willing to discuss this important issue with you.

I prefer being asleep during my surgery. Is general anesthesia available?

People are often confused about anesthesia for cosmetic surgery. They think of being *completely asleep* or *wide awake*. It is not an either-or situation. Rather, a sliding scale of anesthesia is usually involved. Varying amounts of intravenous medications are used, depending on the patient's needs. This allows for many levels of anesthesia in between the extremes of total wakefulness or complete sleep. You may have a deeper level of anesthesia if you prefer. With a combination of local injections and i.v. medications, you feel no pain and remain anxiety-free during surgery. You should discuss anesthesia with your surgeon before the operation. Your surgeon and you can ensure that you get anesthesia that is best for your needs and preferences.

Who gives the anesthesia? Is it the surgeon or an anesthesiologist?

This varies from procedure to procedure. In simpler and shorter operations the surgeon may give the anesthesia. With longer procedures, many surgeons use nurses specially trained to administer anesthesia. Some surgeons prefer using anesthesiologists, who are medical doctors like your surgeon, but who specialize in anesthesia.

The extent of your operation, your health status and your specific requirements are factors that are evaluated by your surgeon in the choice of who administers anesthesia.

SURGICAL PROCEDURES

FOUR

Surgery of the Nose

Rhinoplasty (reshaping of the nose) is the most common cosmetic surgical procedure. This year alone, nearly two hundred thousand people in the United States will have rhinoplasties. The nose is so striking a part of the human face, giving it character and stamping individuality onto one's looks, that even the slightest alteration or deviation is visible to all.

Some people wish for a "perfect" or "ideal" nose, assuming the plastic surgeon has the key or knows what will look best. However, preferences in looks are so personally determined that one should not depend on the plastic surgeon for such standards. The surgeon should really be viewed as a *technical and esthetic guide* for someone seeking cosmetic alteration. You yourself must be the ultimate judge of what is right for you.

When to Have Surgery of the Nose

People of all ages have rhinoplasties. Generally, the nose reaches its final size during the late teens, and this is often the best—but not the only—time for surgery.

People in their twenties, thirties, forties and beyond come for consultation. Most rhinoplasties are done on people in their late teens and early twenties, but many patients have put off surgery for many years—even into their forties and fifties.

Older people constitute a distinct group. They have usually been contented with their noses until they've noticed one of the inevitable signs of advancing age: the drooping that occurs at the tip of the nose. The request is usually for the tip to be lifted. In a sense, then, the older person doesn't seek to change the way he or she looks, but wishes to look as he or she *once did*.

There is no absolute "right time" for a rhinoplasty. The important thing is that the time be right for you!

Your Consultation

During your consultation, you should state what you dislike about your nose. Your surgeon will ask you about your past medical history to determine if there is any medical reason why an operation should not be performed. There follows a physical examination of your nose. Your physician will note the size and shape and skin texture of your nose and face and will make an esthetic and medical assessment. He or she will attempt to determine your ability to breathe in an easy, unobstructed manner. It is essential that any breathing problems come to light. No cosmetic alteration should ever be made at the expense of breathing! You should get a thorough examination of your inner nose and of your capacity to breathe freely. Any existing problem can be corrected at the same time.

What Exactly Is a Nose Job?

A rhinoplasty involves refining and changing the underlying structures of the nose to allow a redraping of the overlying skin. In order to explain how this is accomplished, it is helpful to have some understanding of the basic anatomy of the nose.

The nose is supported at the bridge by two nasal bones, which are attached to the other bones of the face *(see photograph on facing page)*. As we move down the length of the nose, the tissue beneath the skin is cartilage rather than bone.

Basic Anatomy of the Nose

Over these structures lie muscle and a subcutaneous layer of fat. Skin covers all this. Thin skin tends to reflect the subtleties of the underlying cartilage, whereas thick skin obliterates them. An analogy would be to imagine a pencil standing on its eraser, with its point upward. If you drape a sheet (thin skin) over the point, the point will be easily delineated through the sheet. If, however, you drape a quilt (the equivalent of thick skin) the point will be blunted.

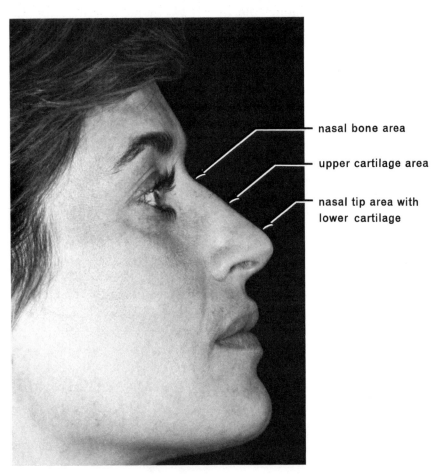

nasal bone area

upper cartilage area

nasal tip area with lower cartilage

The anatomy of the nose.

Two areas of the nose are reshaped in a rhinoplasty—the top and the tip. These two areas are in delicate balance, and the transition between them determines a natural-looking nose or a caricature. The usual request in a rhinoplasty is for "refinement" of the nose, and the balance between the parts is essential for best cosmetic results.

Usually incisions are made through the nostrils, where the scars will remain out of sight. An opening is made in the roof of the nasal bones. With very sharp instruments, the nasal bones are cut at their juncture with the other bones of the face. They can then be moved to close the roof to make the nose narrower and less prominent. The septum (the wall between the nostrils) can also be reduced in height at the middle part of the nose.

The tip is approached in a variety of ways, depending upon the thickness of the overlying skin and the kind of changes to be made. It may be shortened or raised to add the appearance of youth.

The basic concept, then, is a restructuring of the underlying components of the nose and a redraping of the overlying skin. This makes the nose either narrower, or less protuberant, or less bulbous at the tip, and so on. The exact procedure depends on the specific esthetic problem and requirements.

These surgical techniques are constantly being refined and improved. Years ago, with less-advanced techniques, cosmetic change was often obtained at the expense of breathing. Many patients ended up with smaller, more shapely noses, but they had difficulty breathing. This should no longer be the case. If a correction is needed to improve breathing, this can be done during surgery. There should never be a sacrifice of comfortable and natural breathing for esthetics.

Anesthesia for Nose Surgery

As we have described in Chapter Three ("About Anesthesia"), techniques are available today that allow for a painless and anxiety-free operation. As with the surgery itself, your needs should serve as the yardstick in choosing which kind of anesthesia will work best for you. The depth of anesthesia and the type of agent used are adjusted as needed to make for a smooth operation.

When administered by trained professionals, anesthesia is safe. With a healthy and cooperative patient, there are extremely few complications. If you have any questions about anesthesia, discuss them with your surgeon. Simply knowing what to expect before entering the operating room can be very helpful.

Before the Operation

On the morning of the operation you will check into the facility and should meet the people who will be part of your surgical/medical team.

You will be made comfortable with a mild sedative a few hours before your surgery. After an intravenous catheter is inserted into a vein in your arm, you will be ready for your surgery.

The Operation

You are pleasantly sedated and enter into a dreamy state. You will be wheeled on a stretcher into the operating room and will be asked to slide onto the table. The operation will proceed as we have previously detailed. After the procedure the nostrils may be packed, and the nose is covered with strips of tape and a small splint. This nasal splint reduces swelling and allows your newly fashioned nose to heal in the properly aligned position.

After the Operation

Immediately after the operation you may feel drowsy, but this will wear off quickly. Some patients spend the first day at home, while others prefer to remain in the hospital for a short time. At first there will be some stuffiness of the nose. If your surgeon has placed nasal packing within the nostrils (this is becoming less common), you may not be able to breathe through your nose. This may be uncomfortable, but not painful.

The first 24 hours are usually spent in bed with the head elevated on pillows. This is to reduce swelling. After a few hours, liquids may be taken by mouth. This is especially helpful if your nostrils have been packed, since breathing through your mouth may cause drying of your tongue and palate. Medication for pain may be taken if necessary, although most patients feel very little discomfort.

Twenty-four hours after the operation, most people are eating regularly and experience minimal pain. Any discomfort during the recovery period is most noticeable during the first 24 hours. After that, healing proceeds quickly.

The nasal splint usually remains in place for 5 to 7 days. There is no need to remain confined to your home. Indeed, many patients appear in public, feeling little or no concern about being seen with the splint.

The removal of the splint is a major event for both you and your surgeon. Though your nose is not yet in its final form, the dramatic change will be evident. Some slight swelling will obscure the most subtle contours, which will appear later. The important thing to remember is that you've had surgery. This involves manipulation of bone, cartilage and skin, and the response to any surgery is always some swelling. This is completely normal and should not concern you. The swelling will recede over the following few weeks and subtle changes will occur over that period of time. The nose will become thinner and more refined over the course of one year. These changes are so gradual as to be barely noticeable, but were you to have photographs taken every three months during the first postoperative year, the differences could be discerned.

Most patients have minimal discoloration and swelling about the nose and eyes. If this should occur, it is temporary.

With the removal of the nasal splint, most patients return to work and to regular activities. There are, however, some limitations:

You should not engage in active sports for 4 to 6 weeks following surgery.

You should not forcefully blow your nose for a few weeks; this could cause bleeding.

There should be no forceful manipulation of the nose.

During the postoperative period, avoid wearing heavy eyeglass frames that sit on the bridge of the nose. You may find it easier to tape your glasses to your forehead for some period of time each day. This relieves the bridge of the nose from having to support the glasses.

An occasional sneeze is probably inevitable, but you should remember to sneeze with your mouth open for the first few weeks following surgery. This allows air to be expelled through the mouth and not the nose, lessening the chance of a nosebleed.

Bending is permitted, but you should keep your head at a level above your heart. Keeping your head down may cause nasal congestion and a nosebleed during the first few postoperative weeks.

If your nose bleeds, there is no cause for alarm. Lie back with your head tilted, and the bleeding should stop. Do not forcefully squeeze or manipulate your nose. If for some reason you don't know what to do or have a question, *call your surgeon!* This is not an intrusion!

The timetable for healing varies from patient to patient, depending on the kind of surgery and your own healing capacities. You may expect to have some minimal stuffiness of the nose for the first three weeks. This tapers off gradually. Again, the point to remember is that surgery causes some temporary swelling. Flaking of the skin and alteration of skin lubrication may occur. Some time must pass for this to subside.

After approximately six weeks you will have gone through the major portion of the healing process. Afterward, your nose is neither abnormal nor weak. A persistent myth says that after nose surgery the nose is especially vulnerable to being broken. This is not true.

There is one other precaution. For about six months after surgery, you should cover your nose with an effective sun-blocking agent while in direct sunlight during late spring or summer. The sunblock should not be just the ordinary commercial preparation obtained in any pharmacy—it should contain, in addition to para-amino benzoic acid (P.A.B.A.), either zinc oxide or titanium dioxide. This is the whitish material you have often seen on the noses of lifeguards. Various products are available in cosmetic form, so the screening agent need not be displayed in an obvious way. This mixture blocks *all* sun from contact with the skin of your nose. That skin has not yet returned to normal and will burn and swell easily if so exposed.

The postoperative period is a very important one psychologically. With the removal of the nasal splint you finally get to see the long-awaited results of an important step in your life. Most patients express delight at first seeing their new nose. Any postoperative discomfort is quickly forgotten, and most people seem amazed when gazing into a mirror. Even though the healing process is not yet complete, the important profile change is quite apparent. The nose becomes so much the focus of attention that most patients don't notice the minimal swelling around the eyes and nose.

It is perfectly normal to spend a great deal of time viewing your new profile. After all, your entire life was spent with the old one. The new look takes some getting used to. But it is striking how quickly most patients forget their preoperative profile. This becomes very evident when they view their preoperative photographs only a few weeks after the surgery. Of course, a person's willingness to accept, or psychologically integrate, the new look is greatly enhanced if he or she is satisfied with the results. And when a patient has been motivated, has had realistic expectations of surgery, and has discussed all important issues with the surgeon, genuine satisfaction is the rule.

About Change

The change in appearance brought about by nose surgery is more dramatic than that by any other cosmetic facial procedure. In our experience, the vast majority of rhinoplasty patients are extremely happy with the change. This is evident from the moment they first view their newly shaped noses when the nasal splint is removed. Patients often feel euphoric about the change in their appearance. Most patients feel that an unflattering cosmetic flaw has been removed. The new nose is usually smaller, more shapely, and more harmonious with the other features.

In only a few weeks, most patients feel their new look is part of their permanent self-image. Most seem to forget how they looked before surgery!

There is another interesting and important aspect of change you should know about. A recent study* has found that rhinoplasty patients not only feel better about themselves after having had surgery, but *other people* perceive them in more positive ways, too. This study clearly indicates that esthetic surgery—in particular rhinoplasty—enhances physical attractiveness. The study shows that after a rhinoplasty, patients are perceived by others as more friendly, self-assertive, intelligent, and likable.

Possible Complications

While rhinoplasty is a safe procedure, there is always some risk associated with surgery, though trained personnel in the operating room minimize this. Surgery of any kind requires care, great skill, and attention to surgical and medical details.

Infection is possible where an incision has been made in bodily tissues. The rate of infection in rhinoplasty is very low, and with modern antibiotics, there is no reason to be concerned.

Minor nosebleeds may occur during the first postoperative days. They should not cause alarm and can be treated by tilting the head back. After ten days, such occurrences should cease.

Sometimes a postoperative patient may have decreased sensation at the tip of the nose. This is due to the disruption of some

* "Esthetic Surgery: Effects of Rhinoplasty on the Social Perception of Patients by Others." Thomas F. Cash, Ph.D., and Charles E. Horton, M.D. in *Plastic and Reconstructive Surgery*, Volume 72, Number 4. October 1983 Williams & Wilkins Co., Baltimore, Md.

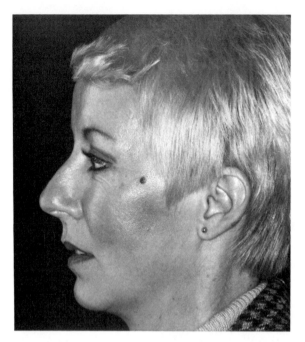

Before rhinoplasty.

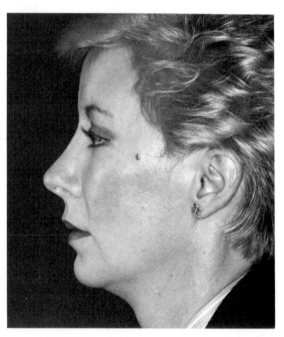

After rhinoplasty.

minor nerve fibers in the superficial skin. There is nothing to worry about; normal sensation will return.

Very rarely, a patient may notice a decreased sense of smell following surgery. This is not because the nerves responsible for smelling have been disturbed. Those nerve tracts are nowhere near the site of the surgery. Rather, this rare problem is caused by swelling of tissues within the nose. As time passes, all will return to normal.

About Unsatisfactory Results

With an experienced surgeon and a realistic patient, the chances of unsatisfying results are small. Recall the case of Roger L., who wanted to look like Paul McCartney. Had a surgeon tried to satisfy his wish, the patient would doubtless have been thoroughly dissatisfied with the results.

Occasionally a patient may be dissatisfied with a rhinoplasty. Nowadays, the tendency in nasal surgery is toward conservatism, and at times, less than the patient had anticipated is actually removed. In such a case, minor adjustments can be made some months after the initial surgery. Such unsatisfactory results need not be permanent. It pays to wait, because over the course of time the new nose becomes more refined as swelling decreases. The remaining "flaw" may have been nothing but swelling. Remember, your surgeon is as eager as you are for you to be satisfied with your surgical results. Your physician will gladly eliminate any minor flaws or imperfections so that you obtain the best possible results.

Frequently Asked Questions

Am I neurotic because I want a nose job?

There is nothing neurotic or unsound about wanting to appear attractive. Many people have a feature that detracts from their looks, and they may be sensitive about this. If your cosmetic flaw is a real one and makes you self-conscious, if your surgical goals

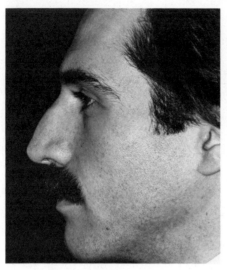

Before rhinoplasty.

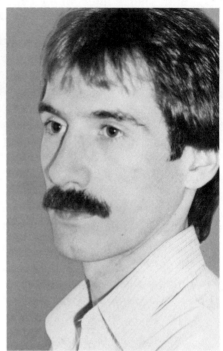

This man underwent surgery to correct a severe nasal septum defect. The result has also made for a pleasing cosmetic change. Note the subtle contours at the tip of the nose. The three-quarter view is very important in evaluating the nasal contour since it is how others usually see you.

*After rhinoplasty
three-quarter view.*

are reasonable, then rhinoplasty is a sound and healthy desire. A number of studies have clearly indicated that a rhinoplasty, when done at the proper time and for the right reasons, brings about an increase in self-esteem.

Does a nose job change your personality?

Of course not. No personality change follows a rhinoplasty. However, with good results, you will very likely feel better about your looks and your self. This rise in self-esteem may change certain ways in which you interact with others and may lead to other life changes. But your basic personality will be the same.

Will I have that "operated" look?

Years ago, when surgical techniques were less refined, many rhinoplasty patients were left with characteristic noses—the so-called ski-slope look, for example—that were really caricatures of a nose. This should no longer be the case. Newer techniques, better instruments and more experience enable a good surgeon to reshape a nose so it appears harmoniously balanced with your other features. Techniques today involve reshaping of nostrils and other parts of the nose. It is also recognized today that a chin augmentation may help achieve balanced facial harmony. (See next chapter.) Here too it may be helpful to see photographs of your surgeon's work with other patients. They should not appear to have that "operated" look.

Will a nose job improve my breathing?

Many people have difficulty breathing because of a deviated nasal septum. The septum is the internal structure (the wall) that separates the right and left airways inside the nose. This wall is composed of cartilage and bone and is covered by a soft lining. A thorough evaluation of your nose should include an assessment of this structure. During surgery, a correction of this deformity will allow you to breathe more easily. Any changes of the external nose should carefully consider the conditions of the internal structures.

Will a nose job improve my allergies?

No. Allergic symptoms (dripping eyes, sneezing, running nose, etc.) have nothing to do with the size or shape of your nose. If, however, you have chronically congested nasal passageways or sinuses, and a deviated nasal septum causes added difficulty in breathing, a correction of this defect may make drainage of the sinuses easier and alleviate the congestion. But your allergy will be unaltered.

How much does a nose job cost?

The cost of any surgical procedure varies from one location to another and from one surgeon to another. At the present time, in New York City, nose surgery costs between $1,500 and $4,000, depending on the extent of the surgery.

Is a nose job covered by health insurance?

Generally, cosmetic surgery is not covered by health insurance policies. However, if some portion of your nose surgery is for repair of a deviated septum or any problem causing difficulty in functioning (for instance, a severely deviated septum may impair free breathing), the portion of the operation and hospital or clinic costs directly related to the correction of the defect may be covered by your health insurance. As always, you must read your health insurance policy carefully to learn which procedures are covered by your plan. Your nose surgery, if done by a licensed physician, is a legitimate medical deduction on your income tax return.

Will my nose be as strong after surgery as it was before the operation?

Yes. After your nose has completely healed it will be as strong as it was before surgery. There is no residual weakness or vulnerability of the nose after the surgery. There is no reason to change your life style after a rhinoplasty:

How long will it be before there are no traces of surgery?

Usually, by the end of the second postoperative week there is no noticeable swelling of the nose. Any discoloration is usually gone by that time also. There does remain a very slight and barely noticeable swelling that will slowly subside over time. Your newly shaped nose will become more refined over a period of months. It takes nearly a year for the final look to be attained. If you were to see serial photographs of yourself taken every few months during the first postoperative year, you would notice gradual and subtle refinements taking place as the nose matures. But for all practical purposes, there is no noticeable swelling by the end of the second postoperative week.

When is the best time of year for a rhinoplasty?

There is no best time of year for nose surgery. You want to have your surgery when you can have at least two weeks for recovery and rest after the operation. This is the only important consideration about time of year.

Will I have scarring?

In any surgery, wherever an incision is made, there is a resulting scar. With cosmetic surgery of the nose, all incisions are usually made within the nostril so that no scar is visible.

How long should I remain in the hospital after nose surgery?

Most surgeons recommend that you remain overnight at the facility where the surgery was done. This is to ensure that you are under observation should there be any postoperative complications.

If I don't like some part of my new nose can it be changed?

When a patient dislikes some aspect of his or her new nose, it is usually minor. Most postoperative changes can be done in the surgeon's office with local anesthesia. If there is some minor postoperative flaw, do not be surprised if *your surgeon* points it out and suggests that it be reshaped some months later.

What if the surgeon removes too much?

This is a very rare complication. As a rule, when a patient is dissatisfied with the result he or she feels the surgeon removed too little nasal profile. However, if too much was removed, the nose can be rebuilt some time later.

I'm 14 years old. Some of my friends have had their noses "done." I'm not sure about mine. Should I have a nose job or should I wait?

You should have surgery for yourself and yourself only, not to please anyone else or to feel part of the group. A good general rule is to have surgery only if you can tell yourself, "I want this operation even if no one but me ever knows I had surgery."

There is another consideration: At 14, your face may not have completely matured. In time, your features may broaden, and your nose, which appears large now, may look more harmonious with your other features. It makes sense to wait a few more years before seriously considering nose surgery.

I'm getting married in six months. I've never told my fiancé about my nose job. Should I tell him before we get married?

If your relationship is an open and honest one, letting your fiancé know about your surgery should not matter. Hopefully, more than cosmetic considerations brings you together, and your fiancé would not think less of you because you've had nose surgery.

This question relates to the case of *JOANNA P.*, who became upset and anxious during her pregnancy because she had never told her husband about her rhinoplasty. Her nose surgery (along with that of her sister and mother) had been done before she met her husband. As her pregnancy progressed she grew increasingly anxious, fearing her child would be born with the same large nose she herself had as a youngster. Her fear escalated to the point where she imagined her husband would be angry and disillusioned with her and would love her less. Realizing her fears were getting out of hand, she talked with a good friend who finally advised her to get psychological counseling.

DR. RUBINSTEIN:

> *JOANNA P.* met with me for a consultation. In a few sessions she felt better and was able to reveal her secret to her husband. She came to realize that her self-esteem was low, since it had taken very little to make her feel she would be unloved and unlovable. She continued in psychotherapy, learning much more about herself. Eventually, she felt more confident and better about herself.

Although surgery had been successful, for Joanna P. it had not eradicated the bad feelings and poor self-esteem she had harbored for many years.

I have hay fever. Can I still have nose surgery?

Hay fever itself does not preclude nose surgery. However, the allergic symptoms must be under control before having surgery.

I have asthma. Can I still have nose surgery?

Asthma can be a distressing—and sometimes life-threatening —condition. Asthma does not stop one from having nose surgery, but the condition must be well under control before the operation.

I want my 14-year-old child to have her nose done, but she isn't interested. How can I convince her that she will be better off with a smaller nose?

If your daughter is happy with her looks it makes little sense to try to persuade her to have surgery. In fact, you may unwittingly foster in your child a poor self-image of herself. Don't pressure her into surgery. Patients who have surgery to please or placate a parent or spouse are rarely satisfied with their results. The entire matter becomes less one of achieving realistic cosmetic results than a battlefield for a host of emotional issues. If your daughter truly has a *significant* cosmetic problem, she may discover it as she gets older. The motivation for cosmetic surgery must come from the *patient*, not from family members.

My 17-year-old son wants a rhinoplasty. He insists his nose has a bump he dislikes. Our friends and relatives see nothing wrong with his nose; nor do his friends. What can we do?

This is a complicated issue. We sometimes encounter a patient who thinks he or she has a cosmetic defect where there is none or where the defect is quite insignificant. Often this person is harboring bad feelings about himself, but the feelings have become centered on a particular feature. This is often the nose, but it can be any feature of the face or body. The person may become obsessed with his imagined or exaggerated flaw, feeling that if only it was corrected life would be fine. It makes more sense for this person to deal with inner conflicts than with changing some outer feature.

If your son speaks with a psychiatrist, he may begin to acknowledge his dissatisfaction with problems deeper than his nose, which may merely symbolize more distressing emotional concerns. The first step may be to consult with a plastic surgeon. If your son has no real cosmetic flaw that requires surgery, the surgeon will corroborate your stand. This could be very helpful in convincing your son that his real problems are deeper than his nose.

My fiancée is an attractive woman but she has a large nose. I'd love for her to get it fixed . . . and I'd pay for the surgery. But she never mentions it and I'm not even sure she thinks it's large. How should I bring the subject up? Am I wrong for wanting her to look better?

There's nothing wrong with wanting your fiancée to look her best. But you may be dealing with deep personal issues here—both in yourself and in your fiancée. Assuming the relationship works well, why would you want her to change her nose? If she has never mentioned it—nor ever even hinted about it—you may assume she is perfectly happy with her looks, despite what to you is a cosmetic flaw. Motivation for surgery should come from the patient—not from anyone else! If she has no wish to change her nose, then you would be asking her to change her looks for *you* and not for herself. Even if she consents, you may be inviting trouble. Having one's looks changed for someone else may bring on resentment and recriminations. If your fiancée were to express a dislike for her nose—or even hint about it—it would be likely she would want you to help her make the decision to have surgery. But until she makes such an overture, you might best explore your own motivations for thinking of this issue as your marriage date approaches.

My 16-year-old daughter insists that the money we were going to spend to send her to camp should instead be spent on a nose job. I think she's too young to make a decision that will affect the way she looks for the rest of her life. Am I wrong?

First, is it the money or the surgery you find objectionable? They should be separate issues.

There is no absolute right or wrong in this situation. Any decision about surgery is influenced by a number of factors. Is there a significant cosmetic flaw that can be helped by surgery? How serious is the flaw? Does it affect your daughter's sense of confidence and well-being? Is it affecting her life? These questions may be difficult to answer objectively, but they must be considered when debating whether or not surgery is appropriate.

It might be helpful for you and your daughter to consult with a plastic surgeon together. Remember, consulting with a surgeon does not obligate you to have surgery. In these meetings you and your daughter may clear up any misconceptions or misgivings about surgery. A good surgeon will evaluate your daughter's situation and help you clarify your differences. It is easier to agree if clear thinking prevails and if you both learn as much about nose surgery as you can.

I resent my daughter's wanting a nose job. I feel she should be proud of her looks. The "family nose" has been good for all of us through the years and I feel she is belittling her origins. Am I wrong?

Right or wrong is not the issue. Your daughter wants to change some aspect of her nose. A common myth is that after surgery the person will look totally changed. Today, surgery attempts to arrive at results with more natural features. Subtle changes may be made to soften features without drastic change. A consultation with a plastic surgeon may be very enlightening.

There are many motives for wanting to change one's nose, but rarely does a person wish to belittle or disavow the family heritage. In our experience, most patients who wish to change their noses feel they would simply look better if this feature were altered. If your daughter does wish to belittle her background, other signs of this intention would, no doubt, have appeared by now.

I'm 23, black and a single woman. I have a broad nose with wide nostrils. I want to retain my basic racial features but want to bring my nose into perspective with the rest of my face. Can plastic surgery help me?

By changing the shape of your nasal bones and by narrowing the tip of the nose you can hopefully achieve your desired cosmetic results.

I'm a 20-year-old man. I broke my nose in a car accident last year and now I've got that "pug" look. Can plastic surgery help me?

Many people with pug noses have been helped by plastic surgery. The septum is an excellent source of tissue to build up the top of your nose. Also, ear cartilage and bone can be used to alter the shape of the top. These possibilities should be explored with your surgeon.

If I have a minor correction a few months after my rhinoplasty, is it considered a separate operation?

Most likely not. Your surgeon will probably view the corrective procedure as part of your overall operation and it will be considered after-care. Most physicians would want you to be as pleased with your results as you possibly can be. After all, part of a physician's reputation will ride on your cosmetic results.

I've been dissatisfied with my nose all my life. I would like to have a rhinoplasty, but I occasionally have severe nosebleeds. Does this make me unsuitable for a rhinoplasty?

You must have your nosebleeds investigated. Most likely, they are not serious. A frequent cause is deviation of the nasal septum. The septum's tissue lining may become dried because of altered air flow through the nostril. This dryness may cause bleeding of the lining. Such deviations of the septum can be corrected at the time external change is made. Other medical conditions can also cause nosebleeds. Your overall medical condition should be completely evaluated before any operation.

I'm concerned I'll be embarrassed by my nasal splint after my nose job. Am I being overly self-conscious?

No. If you choose to appear in public while wearing the nasal splint, expect that some people may stare. It is normal to feel somewhat conspicuous in such circumstances. If this bothers you, plan to remain at home or minimize your public appearances during the first 5 to 7 postoperative days.

I want a nose job but I'm afraid my husband will not accept the change in me and that our relationship may suffer.

As with any other major decision, you and your husband should communicate openly and freely. Part of this communication should include your husband's presence at your consultation. Nasal surgery is not a panacea. If your relationship is troubled, surgery will change nothing. However, in a good relationship, a cosmetic change which makes you feel better about yourself will most likely please your husband too.

I've heard that after a rhinoplasty, some people have a sense of self-alienation; that they can hardly believe it's really them. Is this true?

In our experience, a patient who has had a good working relationship with a surgeon knows what to expect after surgery. Most postoperative patients are delighted when they first look in the mirror and see the new profile. Their basic face is not changed, but their features are brought into better harmony. Most people have a fairly constant image of themselves. A postsurgical sense of self-alienation may indicate that there is an internal, psychological problem which existed prior to surgery.

FIVE

Facial Contouring

In this chapter we will discuss methods of improving facial contours. Two areas of the face can dramatically change your facial contours: the chin and the cheeks.

Sometimes a patient who is dissatisfied with his or her nose is surprised when the plastic surgeon suggests a chin implant in addition to a rhinoplasty. The patient's first response may be, "I've come because of my nose and you're telling me there's something *else* wrong with me!" To understand why a surgeon may make this recommendation, it is helpful to discuss facial harmony.

Facial Harmony

If you look through a beauty magazine you will notice that, though the models look different from one another, there are striking similarities among their faces. Most models have a strong chin and high cheekbones. If you examine the faces in detail, you will probably see that individual noses or eyes or lips are not perfect, but are well balanced. A harmonious overall appearance is more important than a single perfect feature in deciding the person's total look.

Though there are variations in most good-looking people's individual features, the majority of them enjoy *facial harmony*. Most of us know more about facial harmony than we realize, and can easily pick out people whose facial contours match the generally accepted standard of handsomeness or beauty in our society.

When evaluating their own looks, many people focus their attention on a specific feature they dislike. This is often the nose, which may be large or unattractively shaped. But some people with large noses also have very recessed chins. Sometimes a poorly developed chin *alone* may make the nose appear larger than it really is.

The important thing to remember is that *your face must be viewed as a whole*. For instance, a delicate, small nose on a wide, large-featured face would look out of place. When examining your profile, think of your nose and chin (really, all your features) as a unit requiring esthetic balance. Your nose (or any other feature) is an *integral part of your face*. It is not an isolated feature. This concept of facial harmony is important when evaluating your face for any cosmetic change.

Studying Your Facial Contours

Medical-grade photographs are essential tools for studying your features to determine their contours and harmony. Whether you consult with a surgeon because you dislike your nose or because you think your chin is recessed, photographs should be taken frontally and in profile. Using these pictures, the surgeon can pinpoint your problem. Then, by altering the photographs, the physician can approximate how you will look after surgery. Examining these photographs with your surgeon gives you the clearest idea of which cosmetic changes would be most appropriate for you.

The photographs allow you to perform an important test. Your surgeon may take two identical photographs of your face in profile. He will cut the bottom of one photo away. The bottom section of the cut photo shows only your chin. This can then be placed over the other photograph and moved forward and backward. In this way, by sliding the superimposed photograph of the chin in either direction, you may place your chin in the position you think is most appealing. This position is then marked. The disparity between the extent of your actual chin and the chin position you feel is preferable can be underscored by this simple exercise. This may be the first time you have ever noticed such a facial imbalance. Often, after performing this exercise, patients realize it is the *recessed chin* which gives the impression of a large nose, not necessarily the nose itself.

This exercise allows you to contribute in an important way to the final results you want to achieve. We have found that some patients become anxious about having a *recessed chin* pointed out to them when they have come because of a *nose problem*. It can make someone feel that he or she is not in control of what is occurring in the consultation. With this exercise, however, the patient quickly grasps the surgeon's point about the chin and becomes involved in making the choice about his or her new profile.

Medical-grade photographs are also used to study the cheekbones. There is another way of demonstrating the final results when considering a cheekbone augmentation. Your surgeon may fashion the intended cheekbone augmentation from a quick-drying rubber compound used for dental impressions or from stage make-up. By applying this material over the cheekbones and then looking in a mirror, you may see an approximation of your expected results after surgery.

Having Your Chin Augmented

Chin augmentation requires an operation, but it is not complicated surgery. This procedure can be done at the same time as a rhinoplasty, or it is done separately for those whose cosmetic problem is solely a recessed chin.

The operation requires the surgical placement in the chin area of an implant of the size decided upon by you and your surgeon. Currently, most surgeons prefer using a silicone rubber material.

These implants come in many sizes, shapes and consistencies. In special cases they may even be custom-made by your surgeon.

The implant is inserted through an incision at the bottom of the inside of the lower lip. Some surgeons prefer making the incision under the chin. The unit is inserted beneath the skin, fatty tissue and muscle, and fits against the jaw. Only a small space is made for the implant, insuring that it does not move during the healing period.

During the first few postoperative days, there may be some discomfort in the region of the jaw, but there should be no pain. Patients often refer to the discomfort as a sense of tightness, which is reasonable because the overlying tissues are being slowly stretched over the implant. There is some minimal swelling around the jaw for a few weeks after the operation. This swelling is minor and barely noticeable to anyone but the patient. Sutures are removed after about one week. If the incision was made through the inside of the lower lip, there will be no visible scar. If the implant was inserted through the skin under the chin, the small scar will fade in time.

There are few complications associated with chin augmentation. The most frequent one is the chance of infection. This is infrequent, but if it does occur, the implant may be removed and then reinserted at a later time.

Most patients receiving chin implants are extremely pleased with their results. Augmenting a chin may dramatically improve a patient's appearance by improving facial harmony. It is commonly observed that a strong chin and high cheekbones convey a sense of beauty, even though other features are not perfect.

Reducing the Size of the Chin

Some chins are too prominent. Patients can observe this by means of the manipulation of photographs described in the previous section. Sometimes x-rays are helpful. When excess bone in the chin is the problem, it can be removed. The surgical approach in this operation is through the mouth. The soft tissues are lifted from

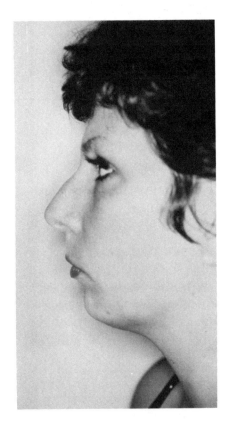

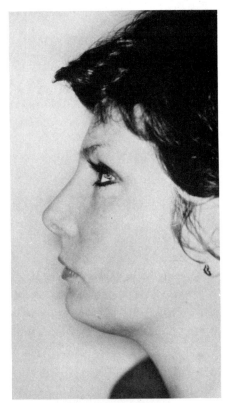

Before operation.

After rhinoplasty and chin augmentation.

This patient initially requested a rhinoplasty. After a consultation, however, she realized that her receding chin was also a major cause for her lack of facial harmony.

the jaw bone in the chin area, and the excess bone is reduced in size and reshaped. In time, the overlying soft tissue shrinks into position around the newly shaped chin.

There are other surgical procedures that move the jawline forward or backward to improve both appearance and the patient's dental bite (occlusion). Such surgery is complicated and is not usually considered strictly cosmetic.

Cheek Augmentation

After you and your surgeon have used soft rubber to demonstrate your new cheekbones, you are ready for a cheek augmentation. As with chin implants, there are many standard-sized silicone materials available on the market. The operation involves the insertion of the properly sized and shaped implants beneath the skin, fatty tissue and muscle so they fit against the cheekbones.

This operation is usually performed through the mouth. The incisions are made at the junction of the inside of the upper lips with the gum. Tunnels are surgically made leading under the soft tissues of the cheek area. The pocket for the implant is precisely fashioned so the implant will remain in its proper position. Some surgeons prefer to fix the implants in place with suture material.

The recuperative period after the operation is short. The patient must be careful not to move his or her facial muscles too strenuously. This is to avoid displacing the implant before healing has occurred. The usual sensation reported by patients is a sense of tightness in the area of the implants. Again, this is due to the stretching of the overlying soft tissues. Complications are minimal and infrequent with this procedure. Displacement of the implant is the one most frequently reported.

A nerve to the upper lip and front teeth is located in this region. The surgeon must take care not to injure this nerve during surgery. A rare complication of surgery is numbness in the region of the upper lip. This usually disappears with time.

The results of a cheek augmentation can be very dramatic, giving a patient's facial contour a more taut and youthful look. Most patients are pleased with how dramatically their newly acquired high cheekbones improve their looks.

Frequently Asked Questions

I'm a 19-year-old college student. My father said that I should get my chin fixed. It's quite recessed, and I've thought about it but I'm not sure. My father says my chin will be a detriment to me in my business career.

In our society there is an unfortunate association of a "weak-chinned" person with one having little strength of character. Of course, this is a myth. The important consideration is whether or not your chin detracts from your looks and causes you emotional concern. If this is so, then you might seriously consider having a chin augmentation. If not, it is unlikely that your chin will impede you in your career efforts.

I'm concerned about having a silicone implant in my chin. I've heard that silicone can "migrate." Is this true?

The silicone used in a chin augmentation is a firm substance, which cannot migrate. The silicone substance that has, on occasion, migrated is the liquid injectable silicone that is not approved by the Food and Drug Administration for use in the face. Once the firm silicone implant is placed in the tissue of the chin and healing takes place, it cannot migrate.

What happens to the silicone implant after it's placed in my chin?

The implant is placed beneath the soft tissues of the chin and is held against the mandible by the healing process and the overlying muscle. Silicone is a very nonreactive substance. The silicone is recognized by the surrounding connective tissues as foreign; it is not the same as bodily tissue. The surrounding connective tissue encapsulates the silicone implant, holding it where it was inserted. Firm silicone implants have been used in surgery for years. Artificial hip joints are an example of such implants.

I've heard that a chin implant feels strange and that there is swelling at first. Tell me more about it.

The implant may feel strange at first, but this should not surprise you. Imagine that you were going skin diving for the first time and that before the expedition you purchased a skin-diving watch. At first it would feel heavy and cumbersome, but after a while you would not notice its presence on your wrist. Likewise, you will become completely unaware of the chin implant after a while. It is incorporated into the body, on both a physical and a psychological basis. The only difference will be the harmonious and pleasing contour of your new chin.

My girl friend had a large chin. She went through a chin reduction operation two months ago. Her chin is smaller now, but not by much. How come?

Your friend's chin does not yet appear significantly smaller than before the operation because there is still swelling around the jawline. Also, in this operation time is needed for the skin surrounding the newly fashioned, smaller jaw to contract. Six months to a year is necessary for these changes to occur.

My chin was always recessed. I had orthodonture when I was younger, which corrected my bite, but I still have no chin. Do I have to have my jaw moved or can I have a chin implant?

In order to have a more pleasing appearance you may have a chin augmentation without resorting to the more complicated surgery involving the jaw. This will not interfere with your dental alignment, since the chin implant is located outside the mouth and rests against the jawbone, beneath the underlying soft tissues. If you are displeased with your profile and feel a change is worthwhile, you should consult a cosmetic surgeon.

I know a model who had her wisdom teeth removed to heighten her cheekbones. Is this possible?

Yes. Some people, wishing to heighten their cheekbones, have their upper wisdom teeth removed. The underlying bone then reabsorbs to some extent. This allows the overlying cheek to sink in slightly and form a sculpted-looking hollow, thereby heightening the appearance of the cheekbones above. The actual amount of heightening is minimal, but apparently some people feel the extraction of the teeth is worth the effort. In general, we would not recommend this approach to cosmetic change.

How much does a chin augmentation cost? How much does a chin reduction cost?

At the present time, in New York City, a chin augmentation costs between $1,000 and $1,500. A chin reduction procedure costs between $2,000 and $4,000.

SIX

Cosmetic Eyelid Surgery

Your eyes are the most telling feature of your face. Their condition and that of the surrounding skin reveal a great deal about how you feel, since your eyes are affected by your environment, your emotions and your age. Cosmetic surgery of the eyelids (blepharoplasty) is an operation performed very frequently and with excellent results.

What Brings People to the Surgeon?

A frequent complaint heard from patients asking about their eyes is: "People ask me if I'm tired or if I had a good night's sleep. Others ask, 'When was your last vacation?' or comment, 'You should take better care of yourself.'" Generally, the realization that adequate rest and dietary restrictions no longer erase the lines or bags about the eyes brings a person to consult a surgeon.

The Causes of Eyelid Wrinkles and Bags

The skin of the eyelids is the thinnest on your face. It is loosely bound to the underlying muscles. Over the years it is susceptible to many influences.

Your eyeball sits in a bony vault of the skull and is surrounded by protective fat. Both this fat and the eyeball itself are covered in the front by layers of muscle and skin, which form the eyelids. Over the years, the skin of the eyelid begins to stretch as a result of various activities and influences—blinking, squinting, sunburn, wind, cigarette smoke, alcohol and diet.

With age, the skin and muscles of the eyelids lose their elasticity and tone and no longer shrink back after being stretched, irritated or inflamed. The underlying fat may then push forward, unrestrained by the weakened muscle and stretched skin. This can produce a puffy appearance of the eyelids, or bags. The stretched skin of the upper eyelid may droop, while the skin of both upper and lower eyelids forms lines which deepen with time. The puffy, stretched look makes for a dissipated or worn appearance.

Some people have a genetic tendency toward puffy eyes. Because of too much fat beneath the skin and muscle, they have always had bulges or pouches. This condition has little to do with aging, although as time goes by it may become more prominent. Some people use skin toners and cosmetics to remove evidence of shadows and folds. These may work well in the early stages, but they eventually lose their effectiveness.

Bagginess of the lower eyelids, deepening of crow's-feet, and loose, wrinkled eyelid skin are usually the early signs of the aging face. The eyelids, because of their constant moving and stretching as well as their thin skin, may show aging before other facial features.

When to Have Cosmetic Eyelid Surgery

There is no single best time for eyelid surgery. The decision when to operate is based on the presence of a cosmetic problem that concerns the patient. One's decision to no longer have old or tired-looking eyes is the main determinant of timing. People of all ages elect to undergo cosmetic eyelid surgery. Occasionally teenagers with genetic bagginess of the lids request blepharoplasty. This operation is performed on people from their teens to their seventies.

When requesting eyelid surgery, you are not seeking to change your looks. You wish to restore a youthful look that you may feel you have lost.

There is a special group of people (usually older) who require blepharoplasty for medical rather than cosmetic reasons. Their aging upper eyelids form a fanlike redundancy of skin, which droops downward. In extreme cases the eyelid skin droops enough to obstruct vision. These people require blepharoplasty.

As with any cosmetic surgical procedure, you should avoid an operation if there has been a recent major change or emotional turmoil in your life.

> *SUSAN B.* was a 34-year-old recently divorced woman who came for a consultation because she was concerned about how old she looked. She singled out her eyes as being responsible for this. When I examined her it was clear that she had some minimal fine lines on her eyelids, which were normal for someone her age. The eyelid area is one of the first areas of the face to display signs of aging. I have seen many patients with such early complaints. For Susan B., the beginning fine lines about her eyes were the focus for an overwhelming obsession about aging. Technically, only minor changes could be achieved, leaving Susan B. with much the same appearance.
>
> Because of her recent divorce and uncertainty about her future, Susan B. was overly concerned about aging. In my estimation, she was not a good candidate for surgery at that time. She really wanted more than her eyes changed. In my view, her problems were more emotional than surgical.

Susan B. was dissatisfied with things since her divorce. She had gone through a major emotional upset in her life and was trying to deal with her turmoil through surgery, as though all of life's unpleasantness could be corrected with a scalpel.

In any consultation for blepharoplasty, your surgeon should ask about emotional problems. The surgeon may have to shift gears if he or she feels there is a significant emotional problem that could possibly get in the way. The surgeon may even feel that a consultation with a psychiatrist is in order. This does not mean the surgeon feels you are "disturbed," but rather means that he or she feels you could benefit by exploring your motivation for surgery. Any intended surgery may always be done at a later time.

How Is Cosmetic Eyelid Surgery Done?

In this operation, the weakened excess skin and stretched muscle of the eyelid are removed. The fat protruding from behind the muscle and skin is also cut away. This gives an appearance of smooth, crisp folds to the upper lids and removes the pouches below the eye.

The following photographs and explanation should make the operation clear.

The incisions are sutured with delicate silk or nylon sutures.

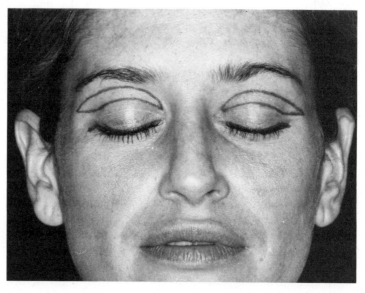

The eyelid incisions. Before the blepharoplasty procedure the amount of skin to be removed from the upper lids is marked with indelible ink. During the surgery the excess skin within these markings is removed. Any excess muscle and protruding fat are also removed. The edges of skin of the upper lids are then sutured together so that the line of the incision falls in the natural fold of the eyelid and is well camouflaged.

There is no such thing as surgery of the eyelid (or of anything else) that leaves no scar. A very fine scar results, but because of its thinness and its location in the natural creases of the eyelid area, it is so inconspicuous as to be hardly visible.

This operation takes one to two hours, depending on the amount of surgery needed. There are variations for additional cosmetic effects. The surgeon can create a crisp fold in the upper eyelid, even where none existed before. Also, the outside corner of the eyelid can be elevated to change its shape. These cosmetic effects can change the way the eyes look, and can be very flattering.

Anesthesia for Eyelid Surgery

As explained in Chapter 3 ("About Anesthesia") the goal is to allow patients a pain-free and anxiety-free experience. Using intra-

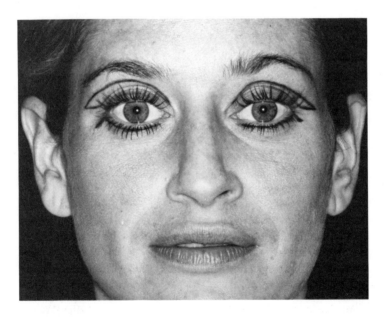

In the lower eyelid the incision is made just below the lashes, along the length of the lower eyelid out to the natural folds at the edge of the eyelid. Any excess fat and muscle are removed. The skin is pulled in an upward and slightly outward direction. Excess skin and muscle are trimmed. The skin edges are then sutured.

venous medication, a twilight sleep is induced. In this state, the patient can respond to commands even though not fully alert. Most surgeons prefer that the patient be able to move the eyelids, making it easier to estimate the amount of excess tissue to be trimmed away. Local anesthetic is injected around the eyelids. These injections block pain, while the intravenous sedative prevents undue anxiety. This combination makes for a *painless* and *anxiety-free* experience. The procedure may be performed with the patient asleep. The choice of anesthesia should be discussed with your surgeon.

Surgery in the Office or the Hospital

Blepharoplasty can be performed in a well-equipped clinic as well as in a hospital. The most important thing is that you receive high-quality care and meticulous attention in the operating suite and during the immediate postoperative period. However, you must have someone near you during the first few postoperative days. You should not return home alone after surgery.

After the Operation

Immediately following the operation you may feel slightly drowsy. This will soon wear off. The first few postoperative hours are best spent in bed, either at the hospital or at the out-patient facility. The first 24 hours should be spent quietly resting on your back. There is very little pain or discomfort. During the second 24-hour period, minimal activities may be started. You can begin eating regularly at this point.

Though there is no pain, there is some minor discomfort. You may have some mild blurring of vision for a few days. This is because your eyelids are swollen after surgery; this leads to minor alterations in the thickness of the tear layer covering the eyeball. Most patients are barely aware that this occurs. The blurring is minimal and disappears as soon as the swelling subsides.

There will be some swelling and perhaps some discoloration of your eyelids after surgery. This is a normal response of tissues to surgery and should not alarm you. The swelling will subside and the discoloration will disappear in 7 to 10 days. You may already have some idea of this if your surgeon has shown you photographs of immediate postoperative patients.

The biggest problem for many patients after blepharoplasty is that they tend to *forget they had surgery!* The postoperative period for most people is so uneventful that they return to excessive activity too quickly. You *must* rest during the first five days following surgery. Here are some do's and don'ts:

No stooping or bending for one week after the operation. Keep your head elevated above your waist. Lowering your head will cause an increase of blood pressure in the eye area and may cause some bleeding into the eyelids. This may also cause more swelling.

For the first five to seven days there should be no vigorous exercise that would raise your blood pressure. This could add to the bruising and swelling already present.

You must wear sunglasses during the early postoperative period. This is not to hide your eyes but to protect the area from dust, wind, sunlight and other irritants.

Avoid rubbing your eyelids. Avoid squinting frequently, and avoid using your eyes excessively (prolonged reading) during the first few days after surgery. The more you move your eyelids, the more you may add to the postoperative swelling.

Sutures are removed three to five days after the operation. Some surgeons replace them with temporary tapes for additional support. By the fifth to seventh day, women can resume using eye makeup. Most patients return to full activity by the seventh to tenth postoperative day. By this time, swelling and discoloration disappear. The fine scars formed by the incision lines will become less visible as the scar tissue matures. Eventually they become inconspicuous.

Possible Complications

While blepharoplasty is a safe procedure, as with any surgery there may be complications. These are almost invariably minor and reversible. They are:

Ectropion. An ectropion is a lifting away of the eyelid from the eyeball. It is usually temporary, but if it remains it can be corrected by minor surgical procedures.

Infection. This is rare in the area of the eyelid.

Blurriness of vision caused by alterations in the amount of tears or in the thickness of the tear layer. As mentioned, this is because of swelling of the eyelid. It is temporary.

Small cysts (milia) in the suture areas. If these occur, they can be easily removed by your surgeon. There may be other minor irritations of the scar tissue as it forms. These are slight and transient. If they occur, discuss them with your surgeon. If necessary, there are medications to minimize these minor difficulties.

Coming Out

Patients are often concerned about what other people may think or say when they return to their daily lives. After blepharoplasty, there is very little dramatic commentary. Friends and relatives may mention how well or refreshed you look. People you haven't seen for some time may even inquire if you've been on a vacation. But essentially you look as you did before, only you appear less worn or dissipated.

Frequently Asked Questions

How much does a blepharoplasty cost?

The cost of this operation varies from area to area and from surgeon to surgeon. As of the date of this book, the operation may

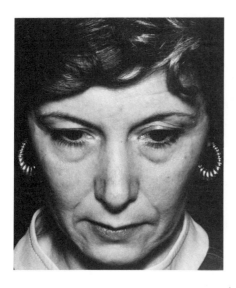

Before blepharoplasty.
Note the excess skin of the
upper eyelids in addition to
the prominent pouches be-
neath the eyes in the lower
eyelid area.

After blepharoplasty. You
can now see the crisp folds
of the upper eyelid. The
pouches are gone. The
patient now looks less tired,
with a refreshed and alert
appearance.

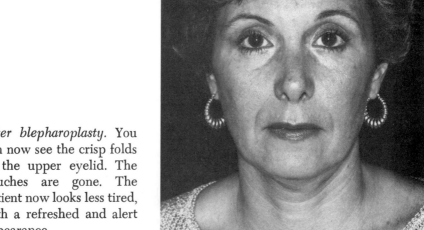

cost between $2,000 and $4,000 in the New York City area. Consulting different surgeons in your area will help you develop a good idea of the range of fees.

Does a blepharoplasty have to be done in a hospital?

No. This procedure, like most cosmetic facial surgical procedures, can be done in your surgeon's office or other out-patient setting. The factors to take into account when deciding where to have your surgery are the quality of the medical team and the standard of operating room and postoperative medical/surgical care.

Will my health insurance policy cover a blepharoplasty?

If your eyelid surgery is done for cosmetic reasons only, your health insurance policy will probably not cover the operation. However, if the operation is done because excess eyelid skin is blocking part of your visual field, the operation is a medical, not a cosmetic procedure. Your insurance will then cover that portion of the operation and hospital cost applicable to the medical need for the operation. However, as a legitimate medical expense, the cost of the operation is a deductible on your income tax return.

Which anesthesia is best for me?

There is no single best form of anesthesia. Some people are uncomfortable with the idea of being put to sleep, while others have no wish to be awake during the procedure. Discuss this with your surgeon before your surgery. As described in Chapter 3 ("About Anesthesia"), a combination of intravenous sedative and local injectable anesthetic is usually used. The degree of sedation varies from patient to patient. The important thing is that you have a *pain-free* and *anxiety-free* experience. The combination of i.v. sedation and local injections ensures this. Some surgeons prefer the patient to be somewhat awake during the operation so that the eyelids can be moved while estimating the amount of tissue to be removed. Here, the surgeon's preference is important.

What about black-and-blue marks? How long do they last?

Black-and-blue discoloration is caused by minor bleeding into the eyelid tissue. This is a common sequel to the operation. The discoloration begins to fade, then turns yellowish, and is completely gone in about three weeks. Within seven days after the operation, you may apply makeup to mask the discoloration. As with postoperative swelling, discoloration is temporary.

When can I return to work?

How rapidly you heal depends on the kind of surgery you have and on your capacity to heal. Most patients return to work within five to seven days after surgery. This is the same for both men and women. Your eyes can function normally at all times, except for some transient blurring that may occur during the immediate postoperative days. It is wise to avoid using your eyes to excess (prolonged reading, distance vision or hours of television) during the first five days after surgery.

I have only slight pouches beneath my eyes. Should I wait until these become more prominent before having surgery?

The main criterion in deciding when to have surgery is how *you* feel about the appearance of your eyes. If you have thoroughly thought out and discussed the surgery and wish to have it, there is no advantage to waiting.

Are the scars visible?

Yes. Your surgeon, by using proper instruments and by properly placing incisions in the folds and creases of the eyelids, will make the scars very inconspicuous. Scars in the eyelid region tend to heal very well, and under normal circumstances no one will see them. However, they are not invisible.

If complications occur, can they be corrected?

Complications are rare. When they do occur (bleeding, excessive bruising, infection, ectropion, excess or changed tearing) they are usually reversible without further treatment. In the rare instances when treatment is necessary (minor surgery, etc.) these complications can be corrected.

My ophthalmologist says he does this kind of surgery. Who is better qualified, my eye doctor or a plastic surgeon?

Some ophthalmologists have been specially trained to do plastic surgery of the eyelids. In some cases, where the drooping eyelids block a patient's vision, the operation is done for medical and *not* cosmetic purposes. However, in order to determine who is more qualified to do this particular kind of surgery, you must inquire about what percentage of the surgeon's practice is composed of *this specific operation.*

My face and neck look wrinkled and sagging. Should I have them done first or should I have my face and eyes done together?

This depends on the extent of work you need on your face and eyes. If the amount of surgery needed is minimal, it makes sense to do both face and eyes in one operation. However, if extensive surgery is required, the two areas should be done separately.

What percentage of eyelid surgery patients are men?

Ten years ago, about five percent of blepharoplasty patients were men. Today, men compose about 50 percent of the patients requiring blepharoplasty in my practice.

Is it true that after a blepharoplasty one eye is raised higher than the other?

This is not true. While human beings are basically symmetrical, there are subtle differences between the left and right sides of your body. Your feet are not exactly alike, nor are your hands, your ears or your eyes. If you see some subtle differences between your eyes after eyelid surgery, it is probably because you are examining your eyes more carefully than before. Any differences between your right and left eyes will no doubt be pointed out to you by your surgeon prior to the operation.

I'm concerned about the younger men in my office and I don't want to fall by the wayside. I've been thinking of having the bags beneath my eyes removed so I'll look younger and be able to compete. Does this make sense?

It makes sense to want to look as well as you reasonably can. If there is a real cosmetic problem detracting from your looks, if your job requires that you look refreshed and vigorous, then it may make sense to consider eyelid surgery. But have realistic goals about it. *Looking* younger doesn't necessarily make you *feel* younger and it certainly doesn't *make* you younger. Your improved looks may help you feel better about yourself and *that* may help your job performance, but no surgery can magically turn you into a young dynamo.

I had a blepharoplasty four weeks ago. Can I sunbathe now?

It is wiser to keep your eyelids out of direct summer sun for about six months after your operation. While the lids look perfectly normal, they are still sensitive, and too much sun may cause swelling and irritation. There are total blocking agents available to protect your eyes from the harmful effects of the sun. It would also be wise to wear sunglasses.

I have glaucoma. Can I still have eyelid surgery?

You may have the surgery if the glaucoma is well controlled with medication. Glaucoma is a disease involving increased pressure within the eye; lid surgery is external and has no bearing on this condition. You must inform your surgeon about the glaucoma and about the medication you take to control it, so that during your surgery no medications will be given that might increase your intraocular pressure.

I've had cataracts removed. May I have eyelid surgery?

Yes, the eyelid surgery has no bearing on your earlier surgery for cataracts. Cataract surgery involves the interior of the eye; a blepharoplasty involves the eyelid only.

I wear contact lenses. Will eyelid surgery interfere with them?

Eyelid surgery will not interfere with your wearing contact lenses. But you should wait about two weeks after surgery before inserting them. The pulling and stretching of the lids involved in inserting the lenses must be avoided. You must wait until all swelling and redness of the lids disappears. Remember too that if you don't wear your lenses for two weeks you must readjust to them gradually once you begin wearing them again.

My wife says I should have my eyes done. Should I do this even if I'm happy with my looks?

Social pressures are a consideration in any decision concerning your looks. However, an operation done to please someone else is usually a mistake. It invites later resentments and possible recriminations. If you and your wife have a reasonably frank and honest relationship, you should be able to discuss your looks and what they mean to both of you. What makes it important to her that you have this cosmetic procedure? Is there an objective problem that makes you look older and causes you some discomfort? These questions must be taken into account—and they must be discussed openly and honestly, without the issue of surgery as a focal point in your relationship. Once a tug-of-war develops, the pros and cons of surgery become more difficult to evaluate objectively.

I have bags under my eyes. I'm 40 years old and I'm a man. I feel funny about going to see a plastic surgeon . . . to me, their patients are all women. I think I'd feel foolish even making an appointment. Can you help me?

Your view of plastic surgery has been commonly held for years. Today more and more men are requesting blepharoplasty operations. Women are not the only ones interested in their personal appearance. Many plastic surgeons today report that from 25 to 50 percent of their blepharoplasty patients are men.

I have bags under my eyes. I've noticed that they seem to be larger and fuller in the morning. An hour later, they've receded. What causes this?

As we age, skin and muscle begin to stretch. When you are asleep the muscles of the eyelid area are at rest. In this condition, fatty tissue pushes forward more readily, and in the morning bulges under your eyes are more prominent.

As you move the eyelid muscles after awakening, the fatty tissue is pushed back, partially reducing the bulge. Late at night or when you are very tired, the bulging will again become prominent, since the muscles of the lids are weakened by fatigue.

I have dark coloring beneath my eyes. This really makes me look tired and dissipated. What causes this?

Some people have a darker pigmentation in the skin of the eyelids. If the discoloration beneath your eyes is caused by hyperpigmentation (too many melanin pigment granules in this tissue) a possible solution is chemical peeling. This involves the application of a phenol solution to the skin. This results in a decrease in the melanin pigment granules of the skin and lightens the skin under the eyes. Chemical peeling will be discussed in Chapter Nine. Also, there are medications that may be applied to lighten the color of the skin. Consult with your plastic surgeon for the best method for you.

How long after my blepharoplasty must I refrain from wearing false eyelashes?

You must not wear eye makeup or false eyelashes in the immediate postoperative period. You must wait until all swelling of the eyelids has disappeared. Any excessive manipulation of the eyelids should be avoided. Usually, patients can resume wearing false eyelashes one week after blepharoplasty.

I'm near-sighted. I've heard that if I have my eyelids done it can improve my vision. Is this true?

This is not true. Near-sightedness (myopia) is caused by certain internal conditions of the eyeball and has nothing to do with the eyelids, which are external to the eyeball and not related to vision. The eyelid protects the eyeball and, by blinking, spreads the tear layer evenly over the eyeball, thus lubricating this delicate organ. The eyelids have nothing to do with the acuity of your vision.

SEVEN

Face-Lift Surgery

What Causes Wrinkles and Sagging?

With age, various changes occur in facial skin. Connective fibers located within the skin layers allow the skin to stretch and then return to its former shape. Over the years these connective fibers decrease and they function less efficiently. The skin cannot easily return to its former position after it is stretched. We all know that a young person who loses 40 pounds may end up with tight skin, while an older person having lost the same weight will then have loose, hanging skin.

With time, these skin changes result in a downcast look of the face, as the skin, the muscles and the fat beneath it begin to droop. The aging face has specific areas that are most likely to be affected by this process. These include the drooping of the brows, the downturning of the nose, the downturned corners of the mouth, the heaviness of the jowls causing the loss of a sharply contoured jaw, the drooping and deepening of the folds running from the nose to the corners of the mouth to the jaw. This facial drooping is the result of ongoing changes in the skin, fat and muscles of the face.

When to Have a Face-Lift

Most people requesting surgical face-lifts are between the ages of 45 and 60, although there are both younger and older patients.

About three quarters of patients are women, and most are frank about their reasons for desiring surgery. "I just don't like looking older." Some patients ask the surgeon to "take a few years off my face." To many people, a distressing feature of the aging face is the sagging, crêpe-like neck. "It makes me look so old!" many patients complain. Many people hope that an operation to rejuvenate their appearance will make them look as young as they feel. As a matter of fact, many people requesting face-lifts say, "Doctor, I'm tired of looking older than I feel!" They often feel that on the inside they are young and vital, but that somehow their appearances are betraying them.

When to have a face-lift is an important question; so is the issue of *when not* to have surgery.

> *MRS. T.*, a 64-year-old woman, was never bothered by the signs of aging. She was an attractively handsome woman who had worked with her husband throughout the many years of their marriage. She had been largely responsible for the growth of their business.
>
> After his death, she became even more involved with the business, working later hours and making new contacts to increase the company's sales. The couple never had children, and now Mrs. T's substantial energies were focused only on the business. She had become a dynamo.
>
> Some months later she came to my office and requested a face-lift, saying, "I have to look younger because of my business."
>
> When I asked her to tell me more about her desire for a face-lift, she hesitated, then stammered uncertainly and suddenly began crying. She admitted she had kept her feelings bottled up during the eight months since her husband's death, and that her entire life now revolved around the business. She said she had not cried about her husband's death—not even once.
>
> It was clear that Mrs. T. had not yet recovered from the loss of her husband. She had funneled her energies into the business rather than deal with this important loss. Though Mrs. T's face

showed signs of aging, surgery would not have been appropriate at that time. The more pressing issue was dealing with the loss of her husband. In a sense, she wanted to turn back her *emotional clock.*

A year later, when she had more fully acknowledged and come to terms with her loss, Mrs. T. had a face-lift with gratifying results.

We occasionally see a patient who requests face-lift surgery when there are only minimal signs of aging. While such cases are rare, they do occur. Some people may exaggerate the first signs of aging. Fearful of getting older, they view the most minor facial crease or change in skin tone with undue alarm.

MISS K. came for psychological counseling after having consultations with four different plastic surgeons over a six-month period. She had requested face-lift surgery, and each surgeon had refused to operate on her. Two had recommended that she seek psychological help. Miss K. was 41 years old. She was an attractive woman with clear skin, pleasing features and a good figure. She could easily pass for a woman in her early to middle thirties. From the moment she walked into my consultation room, it was obvious why the surgeons had refused to operate on her. She was an attractive 41-year-old woman who looked *younger* than her age!

In a few sessions it was clear what had really brought Miss K. to the surgeons' offices. She was unhappy with her life and saw very few prospects for the future. She had been engaged to three different men over the course of fifteen years. All the relationships had ended unhappily because Miss K. had backed out of them, fearful of making a lifelong commitment to any one man. She had always wondered if she might do better.

Now, at the age of 41, having taught high school for nearly twenty years, with no prospects of marriage on the horizon and with her social life meager, she began feeling lonely and unfulfilled. She feared she would never marry; that time was running out for her. This feeling became more pressing when she realized at the beginning of the school term that, if she wished, she could soon retire with a good pension. She began thinking of herself as a spinster and an "old school-marm."

Miss K's problems were emotional and not surgical. She agreed that, rather than continuing her odyssey to more surgeons, she would be better off exploring her emotional problems. She wanted to learn why she had been unable to form long-lasting relationships with men and why she had always wanted to pursue an illusory knight on a white horse.

In another group of patients, the request for face-lift surgery is coupled with important psychological concerns. Occasionally, men request surgery, fearing they will no longer be able to compete with younger men at the office. This must always be evaluated carefully. There are situations where a youthful appearance is vital for job advancement or to maintain one's position. Many men, not necessarily fearful of aging, are afraid of losing their jobs to aggressive, younger men. For them (and for many people), self-esteem is tied to their work lives. They *must* work in order to feel worthwhile, and they need to feel they are successful at their work. These are normal, commonly encountered feelings. Such people may be good candidates for face-lift surgery, provided they are not looking for something unrealistic in the surgery.

Occasionally a patient will have unrealistic expectations about face-lift surgery. A patient may harbor the incorrect notion that a face-lift will not only erase years from his face, but will also turn him into a young dynamo. Unrealistic expectations about the results of facial rejuvenation can only lead to disappointment. A complete consultation will resolve such misunderstandings.

The Consultation

A person requesting a face-lift does not wish to look different, but wishes to look as he or she once did. A usual question the patient has is, "How much better (younger) can I be made to look without looking artificial?" The surgeon must answer this important question to the patient's satisfaction. As with all other consultations for cosmetic facial surgery, the consultation should be viewed as a series of meetings until the patient feels informed and comfortable with the idea of surgery.

Your medical history should be carefully taken. This, along with an examination of your facial configuration, helps the physician form a mental picture of your potential postoperative looks. A surgeon who can convey that picture to you as accurately as possible will make your entire experience more pleasant and satisfactory.

An important aspect of your consultation consists in having preoperative photographs taken of yourself. This may be done either by the surgeon, by a member of his staff or by a medical photographer. Examining these photographs with your surgeon can help you understand *exactly* which area(s) of your face or neck need correction. You can see yourself much more objectively in a photograph when reviewing it with the surgeon. The more objective you can be about your features, the more reasonable will be your expectations of surgery.

As in other consultations concerning cosmetic facial surgery, preoperative and postoperative photographs of other patients are important. These should be photographs of patients your own age, with similar skin tone and thickness, and with similar cosmetic problems. The photographs allow your surgeon to approximate the results you could reasonably expect.

By comparing your own preoperative photographs with those of other patients, you will quickly learn that not all face-lift operations are the same. You may have fullness in the jowls and deepening of the groove from the nose to the corner of the mouth. Another patient may have difficulty in the area of the neck. Each of these problems requires a variation in the surgical approach in order to be corrected. In essence, then, discussing your own photographs with your surgeon allows you to learn which areas and characteristics of *your face* would be most beneficially affected by a face-lift.

A complete medical history is an integral part of the consultation, since many face-lift patients are in the older age groups. Any medical problem can increase the risks of surgery; and all medical problems, no matter how seemingly insignificant, should be discussed with the surgeon.

What Is a Face-Lift Operation?

During a face-lift, sagging layers of muscle and fat will be repositioned and (if necessary) partly removed. The overlying skin will be more tightly redraped over them. Incisions are made as shown in the photographs on the following page and the skin is lifted from the underlying fat and muscle. If excess fat is present, an appropriate amount is removed. This is usually done in the jowl area and beneath the chin. Fat-sculpting in this area can add a sleek, youthful, angular look. If there is sagging muscle, some may be removed too. The muscle may also need repositioning. This adds to the youthful appearance of the face. The skin is redraped over the other tissues and excess skin is removed. The skin is then sutured closed. Fat-sculpting and repositioning of muscle are new advances in facial cosmetic surgery and have added newer dimensions to surgical rejuvenation of the face.

The incision lines and sutures are mostly located within the hair (which need not be shaved) and remain unseen. There is a short portion of the incision line located in front of the ear, which, after it heals, leaves almost no trace. If extensive work is needed in the neck area, a small additional incision is made in the natural fold beneath the chin.

The area where surgical work is done (the neck, mid-face or temple area) varies from patient to patient, depending on the cosmetic problem to be corrected. The operation may take from two to five hours, depending on the extent of work being done.

A Day Before the Operation

About one day before surgery you must have a complete physical examination and tests to ensure that you are in good health. This may be done at your family doctor's office or at the facility where you will have the surgery. You will also be advised by your surgeon to shampoo and shower with a prescribed antiseptic solution for several consecutive days before surgery.

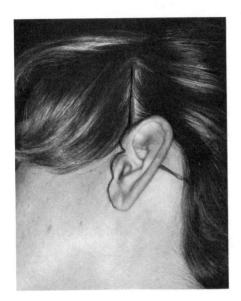 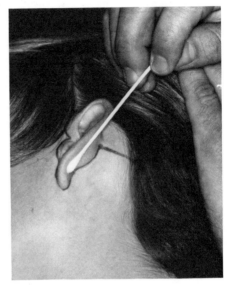

The face-lift incision. The extent of the face-lift incision is shown in these pictures. The usual incision extends from the area in the hairline above the eyes, down in front of the ear, around behind the ear, and out into the scalp.

Before the Operation

Before the operation, an intravenous catheter will be placed in your arm so that medication may be quickly and painlessly administered during surgery. About an hour before the operation you will be given a sedative, which, depending on the amount and type of medication, will make you drowsy or slightly euphoric. As explained in Chapter Three ("About Anesthesia"), you will be relaxed and anxiety-free so that after entering the operating suite there will be very little you will feel or recall.

In the operating room you will be placed on your back with your head slightly elevated. The force of gravity on any excess skin is different in this position from what it would be if you were upright. Because of this, the surgeon is specially dependent upon the preoperative photos to determine where excess skin should be removed.

Your face, neck and hair will be cleaned with antiseptic solution. Then, indelible lines will be drawn where the incisions will be made. Nearly all incision lines will be through the hair. Your hair need not be shaved to do this. It has been learned over the years that shaving the hair is not necessary for sterile operative technique.

After the Operation

After the operation a bulky dressing is usually applied to the face, head and neck. The eyes are left uncovered so vision is not interrupted.

The most important thing to remember is to remain still and quiet. You may be drowsy for a short time after surgery. The next few hours are spent in a recovery area. You should be monitored and supervised by a trained nursing staff. Surprisingly, there is little or no pain after the surgery. If there is *any* pain in the face or neck area you should *immediately notify the nursing staff!* Pain could be an indication of bleeding under the skin, which would require immediate attention. Do not hesitate to report *any* uncomfortable sensations. Some hours after surgery, many people experience a sense of tightness in the face and neck area. This is because of postoperative swelling of the tissues beneath the skin, which press outward against the skin "envelope." This is normal and should not concern you.

You should remain in bed for the first 24 hours following surgery. During this time you will probably be restricted to liquid meals. Most patients elect to stay at the hospital overnight so they can be observed for any possible complications. After the first day, you may gradually return to a solid diet and resume very light activities. The following day, between 24 and 48 hours after the operation, the dressing is removed. It may be replaced by a smaller, second dressing or by nothing at all, depending on the extent of the operation and your condition. If drains have been placed in the incision areas, they too are removed at this time. This is not painful.

All this can be accomplished in a hospital, in a clinic, or at the surgeon's office. Nowadays, there are sophisticated out-patient facilities available for full convalescence. This can be planned before surgery so that you will have the convalescent setting of your choice.

During this time you must rest and remain fairly immobile. There should be no extensive chewing of foods or any vigorous moving of the mouth. This is to allow the area to heal without disturbance.

Bruising and swelling may be present at this time. For the immediate postoperative period some surgeons recommend various dietary regimens to promote healing. Such regimens will vary from patient to patient and from physician to physician.

By day four to eight the sutures in front of your ears will be removed. These are the only areas where the incision lines are visible. In general, all sutures are removed as soon as it is safely possible, to prevent suture marks from forming.

At about day five, your face will still be swollen. Areas of discoloration will persist, but these should not be of concern. At one week, you may shower and shampoo.

After 10 days to 2 weeks the remaining sutures are removed. Most patients are now ready to appear in public with confidence. Of course, the rate of healing depends on your capacity to heal and upon the extent of the surgery.

The following are guidelines for the postoperative period:

Do not apply hair coloring for a minimum of three weeks. Make sure your surgeon gives you the go-ahead before you do so.

Do not bend or stoop so that your head is below the level of your shoulders. This is to prevent any elevation of blood pressure in the face and neck regions and to prevent swelling or bleeding into this area.

You should not engage in vigorous activity or exercise for about six weeks after surgery. Only light activity is permitted until then. This is to prevent an elevation of blood pressure and possible bleeding into the operative site.

You should sleep without pillows and lie on your back during the postoperative period. Forced bending of the neck due to pillows causes tightening of the neck area. Avoid having your chin down, so that you will not cause further postoperative swelling.

Do not use makeup near the incision lines for at least one week.

Avoid sunbathing for at least four months. Remember, the tissues of your face and neck, having undergone surgery, are still sensitive. They will burn and swell easily. When you must

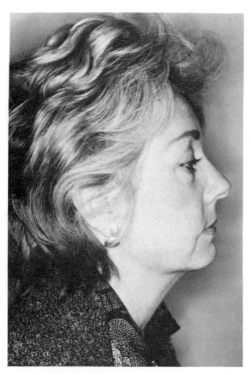 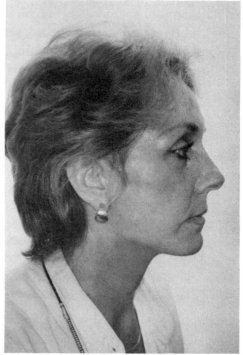

Before a face-lift.   *After a face-lift.*

Note the more youthful jawline and neck area. Operative results are not a mystery! You can see them for yourself in your surgeon's preoperative and postoperative photographs of other patients. (*Photographs courtesy of Vincent DiGregorio, M.D.*)

be exposed to direct sunlight, you should use a protective block containing para-amino benzoic acid (P.A.B.A.) as well as zinc oxide or titanium dioxide. These protective ingredients are available in various commercial preparations manufactured to match natural skin tones. With these blocking agents you may resume outdoor activities about two weeks after surgery. (This does not mean you may bake yourself in direct sun.) Remember, sun and wind are enemies of youthful-looking skin; there is little else that will age and dry your skin as completely as prolonged exposure (when unprotected) to the harsh rays of the sun.

About the Post-Op Blues

Occasionally a patient becomes sad and despondent after surgery. Such a patient may feel bad because one week after the procedure, rather than looking great, he or she finds there is still some swelling and no magical transformation has occurred. This usually occurs because the surgical process was not properly explained to the patient and because not enough time was taken to explore the patient's motivations for and expectations of surgery. This rare occurrence does emphasize, however, the immense importance of good communication between the patient and the surgeon.

In our experience, most patients having face-lift surgery are very pleased with their results. This is so for the immediate postoperative period and thereafter. There is an occasional patient, however, who entertains unrealistic expectations.

MRS. S. was a 62-year-old woman who came for psychological counseling because she was despondent. She had been referred by Dr. Cirillo. Her melancholy had developed slowly over the course of three months. Six months before, she had had face-lift surgery with excellent results. She was elated with her looks the moment she first saw her new face. So were her friends, who were busily arranging to have face-lift surgery themselves. Her good feelings continued for a few months and then she slowly began feeling sad. She had a peculiar complaint. She said, "I've been feeling terrible since my face-lift. It's changed me somehow."

I asked Mrs. S. to tell me more about her life. She had been married for 38 years. Her two children were grown and lived away from her. She and her husband had become distant from each other over the preceding few years. This had been troubling Mrs. S., though she never talked with her husband about it.

Six months before Mrs. S's sixty-second birthday, her husband said she could have face-lift surgery as a birthday present. She was delighted, having expressed interest in having the operation for a number of years. She saw a surgeon in consultation. It was clear that she was a good candidate for surgery. She had some telltale signs of aging that she wished to have eliminated. She did not have unrealistic expectations of the surgery, realizing she would not turn into anyone she was not before the operation—or so she said at the time. The surgery was done with excellent results.

Then, her depressed feelings began building. In the next few sessions it became evident that more had been going on than met the eye. Mrs. S. had viewed her husband's generous birthday gift as a sign that he wanted to revive their earlier closeness. Though the surgery went well and she was pleased with the results, nothing changed in Mrs. S's marriage. She had hoped—unrealistically— that her husband was going to change his attitude toward their marriage. She did not have unrealistic expectations about the surgery. Instead, Mrs. S. was unrealistic about the *meaning* of the surgery. For her, it was a symbol for something else, something she could not have—a closer tie with her husband. The realization that nothing had changed led to trouble.

I pointed all this out to Mrs. S. and she felt somewhat better. But it was clear that she could still get depressed about her relationship with her husband unless something changed in the marriage. I suggested that Mrs. S. take an active role in discussing her feelings and expectations with her husband. She was unsure he would be willing to have such a dialogue, and she felt it would be better if both she and her husband met with me together. Fearful that he would react negatively, Mrs. S. asked her husband to join her in the next session. To her surprise, he gladly complied and agreed that we should have sessions together so the couple could explore their relationship.

Possible Complications

Though face-lift surgery is generally safe, some patients may experience certain complications. Most are not serious and are easily corrected, but you should be aware of them. Complications occasionally occur with the best of surgeons. These professionals are present to see you through this period. The following is a list of possible complications:

Postoperative bleeding. There may be bleeding under the skin that was lifted during surgery. This may result in an accumulation of blood beneath the skin (a hematoma). If this occurs, it is usually small and reabsorbs by itself without further surgical intervention. In the rare instance when the hematoma is larger, an additional procedure may be required to remove the blood from beneath the skin. This procedure, which is not painful, will be done by the plastic surgeon.

Skin slough, a loss of layers of the skin. At times, after surgery, with further swelling, the skin is stretched. There is loss of circulation to this skin, resulting in superficial scar formation. This may require correction at a later date.

Infection. This is also rare and is not a cause for concern. With modern antibiotics, an occasional infection is readily halted and reversed.

Injury to the facial nerve. This is the most potentially serious complication of face-lift surgery. This nerve controls the movement of the facial muscles and runs deep within the muscles and tissues of the side of the face. Bruising or damage to the nerve may cause weakness or loss of the ability to move the affected side of the face. This complication is very rare and is usually temporary. Within weeks the nerve's functioning usually returns to normal. There are a few instances where the damage is permanent.

Numbness. Occasionally, areas of skin remain numb because of the interruption of sensory nerves to the skin. This is usually temporary.

While these complications are few, you should know about them. In our judgment the benefits of face-lift surgery outweigh the occasional complications that may arise, but this is a decision that each person must decide for himself or herself.

Coming Out—What to Expect

You can expect to see dramatic results immediately after your operation. Though there is some swelling, and there may be some discoloration, these will subside over the next two weeks. But the folds, sags and wrinkles of your face are gone, and this is plainly visible the moment your surgical dressing is removed. After one week, swelling recedes and the face begins to regain its normal shape. Some patients are surprised to find that, as the swelling recedes, some very fine wrinkles reappear, which disappeared with the immediate postoperative swelling. But as time passes, the face takes on a more vital and youthful appearance; the cheekbones appear higher, and the face has a crisp, fresh look. As the face-lift matures, you can expect a rested, youthful and vivacious appearance.

By the second to third week after the operation, most swelling has completely subsided. All sutures have been removed. The thin scars in front of the ears will have a somewhat pink appearance, but are easily disguised by makeup. By three months, only your hairdresser will notice these pencil-thin scars.

By six months, the face-lift can be said to have truly matured. You will no longer be surprised when friends and relatives tell you how young or refreshed you look.

Some people are surprised when they receive no dramatic comments from friends. This is not unusual. Remember, the object of the operation is to produce a natural, more graceful and youthful appearance, not to pull back on the skin so tightly that your face seems masklike and artificial.

Frequently Asked Questions

How much does a face-lift cost?

The cost of face-lift surgery varies from one region to another, from one surgeon to another, and depends on the extent of surgery needed. At present, in New York City, the cost of this surgery ranges from $3,000 to $6,000.

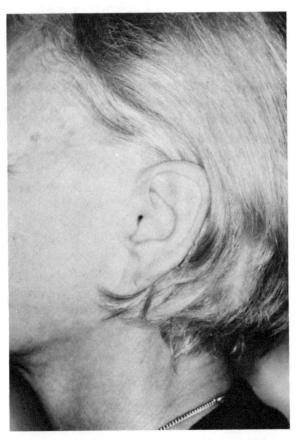

Healed face-lift scar. The only area visible to others is in front of the ear. This picture showing average skin quality was taken one year after operation.

Must face-lift surgery be done in a hospital?

No. Like other cosmetic facial surgery, a face-lift may be done in an out-patient facility or at the surgeon's office. Today, more and more facilities are available for such surgery. They have post-operative recovery areas. The major issue to consider when evaluating having surgery at such facilities is the availability of expert personnel and equipment. A good out-patient facility will have all the necessary equipment and trained professionals to ensure that your surgery will be done in safety and comfort.

How long after my face-lift must I stay in the hospital?

Most surgeons feel that after surgery a patient should be observed overnight. Although this is not mandatory, it is wise, since remaining overnight allows for more careful postoperative monitoring of any possible complications. Most out-patient facilities will make arrangements for an overnight stay.

How soon after my face-lift can I appear in public?

This varies with the extent of your operation, the speed with which you heal, and how you feel about "coming out" before you look your best. You may go grocery shopping and appear in public from about day 3 to day 5 after surgery. Of course, you should take precautions; you must not bend or stoop and should not engage in heavy exercise. You will still be somewhat swollen, but you yourself will be more aware of this than anyone else will be. Generally, most people feel comfortable being seen in public one week after surgery.

Does my health insurance policy cover the cost of a face-lift?

Generally not. This surgery is for cosmetic purposes and is not covered by most policies. However, any such surgery, if done by a licensed physician, is legitimately tax deductible as a medical expense.

If I have a face-lift, will my face then "fall" faster?

No. A face-lift will not stop you from aging, but neither will it increase the speed at which you age and consequently look older.

The operation is a correction that neither speeds up nor slows down the aging process.

How long will the results of a face-lift last?

The rate at which your face ages depends on many factors. Among them are exposure to various elements, such as strong sun and wind, irritants, smoking, excessive alcohol and so on. You may have a genetic predisposition toward looking older or younger. Chronic emotional stress may also take its toll on your looks. However, there is no doubt that once you have had a face-lift you will look younger than if you had not had the surgery.

Consider the following example. If you have face-lift surgery, you will look about ten years younger than your twin sister. The likelihood is that you will always look ten years younger, although you will both age at the same rate.

Will I need another face-lift?

This depends upon the individual patient. Face-lift surgery can turn the clock back but it cannot stop the clock from ticking. How soon you may wish to have your face lifted again depends on many factors: how quickly you age, how well you take care of yourself and of your facial skin, and how you react psychologically to the aging process. However, the benefits of face-lift surgery do not disappear, even though you continue to age as time passes. Today, with newer surgical techniques involving the removal of excess or drooping layers of fat and muscle, the length of time between operations is usually increased.

Should I wait until I really need the operation?

This is a matter of individual choice. It is best to have the operation at a time when the signs of aging become distressing to *you*. Keep in mind that it is more difficult to rejuvenate a much-older-looking person than one who, though showing signs of aging, still has a youthful appearance and whose skin retains a certain integrity and elastic resilience.

How long after surgery must I wait before going into the sun?

First, you must remember that prolonged exposure of the skin to intense sunlight is harmful under *any* circumstances. After face-lift surgery, your skin is extremely sensitive. Most surgeons agree you should remain out of direct sun immediately after surgery. If you wish to expose yourself to the sun you should do so *only* when protecting your skin with *total* sunblocks. These contain, in addition to para-amino benzoic acid (P.A.B.A.), either zinc oxide or titanium dioxide and effectively block *all* rays of the sun. With these sunblocks, you may enjoy the sun.

Will I have any hair loss with a face-lift?

Some loss of scalp hair may occur where the lifting of the skin away from underlying tissues interrupted the hair follicles. Many surgeons go deeper on this portion of the operation near the temples. Some hair is lost because most incisions are placed in and excess skin is removed from the hair-bearing portion of the scalp. However, with newer techniques, hair loss is inconsequential. The very fine scar that results from the operation is easily covered by adjacent hair.

Will a face-lift help my brow wrinkles?

A face-lift will help slightly with the brow wrinkles on the lateral (outer) area of the eyebrow. It can smooth out the vertical wrinkles above the nose, but it does not accomplish either of these very well. Other procedures, such as the brow-lift (next chapter), are more suited for correcting these cosmetic problems.

Are the scars from a face-lift visible?

Cosmetic surgeons try to minimize scar formation and hide scars so they are barely discernible. There are a variety of techniques to do this. Incisions are placed within the hairline, above and behind the ear. There is a small area where the scar will be visible, just in front of the ear. Sometimes the surgeon will make this incision so it falls within the folds of the ear itself, making it even less visible. How well one heals depends on a number of factors. Among them are your skin thickness or thinness, your skin color and swarthiness, and the amount of surgery performed. The resulting scars are pencil-thin, hidden and barely discernible. Scars from face-lift surgery are rarely visible to anyone but yourself and, perhaps, your hairdresser.

Because I'm frequently on and off diets, I tend to lose 15 to 20 pounds and then regain the weight in a few months. Is it best to have face-lift surgery when I'm at my top weight or at my lowest?

This is an important question. First, let's deal with the issue of weight gain and loss as regards the face. Many older patients have excess skin that may form a "turkey-gobbler" neck. They often feel they look better when they have gained weight. This is because they store excess fat in various parts of the face and neck. The accumulated fatty tissue fills out, or rounds out, the skin envelope so there is little excess or hanging skin in this region. What they do not realize is that the extra hanging fat places an additional burden on the already stretched and weakened skin. When this person loses weight, the excess skin tends to hang even more pronouncedly.

While we cannot recommend that you gain and lose 15 to 20 pounds with any frequency, we realize that for many people this seesaw pattern is part of their lives. Therefore, if one were to have face-lift surgery, it would be best to have the operation at a time when the body weight is lowest. With the excess skin hanging, the surgeon may remove a greater amount of it. Should weight be gained at a later time, the now tightened skin will slowly stretch to accommodate the increased amount of fatty tissue collecting beneath. It would be best to remain at your ideal weight without fluctuating.

Is a chemical peel or dermabrasion an alternative to a face-lift?

No. A face-lift will help rid your face of loose, hanging skin and will rid it of certain deep furrows and lines. A chemical peel or dermabrasion (see Chapter 9) is specifically designed to eliminate certain fine wrinkles that cannot be eliminated by face-lift surgery.

Should I have my face-lift and eyelid surgery done together?

This makes sense if you have problems about the eyes and the face and neck area as well. The combination of eyelid and face surgery may be done if the amount of surgery is not too extensive. You should discuss this with your surgeon.

What is the mini-lift?

The mini-lift is minimal surgery with very minimal results. A small incision is made in front of the ear and the skin is stretched back and resutured. This affects the area near the temples only, and ignores the lower face and neck. It is very superficial and does not take into account the various factors involved in the aging face. It may have a place when it comes to fine-tuning a face-lift, but as a *primary* procedure by itself, it is superficial and inadequate.

How many times can a face be lifted safely?

There is theoretically no limitation on the number of times a patient may safely have a face-lift. The procedure may be repeated when the patient's face again takes on a drooping or downcast look. Any muscle needing repositioning can be treated. Excess fat may be removed, and the skin may once again be redraped over the underlying tissues. Excess skin is once again removed.

Is there a minimum or maximum age for a face-lift?

Not really. There are surprisingly young people who have had face-lift surgery because of various skin and muscle problems that made them look older than their true ages. There are people who have face-lift surgery well into their sixties, seventies and beyond.

I want to avoid face-lift surgery. Does it make sense for me to do facial exercises such as grimacing, clenching my teeth and so on?

Such exercises will probably strengthen the muscles of your face but will do nothing to prevent the signs of aging. Remember, the more animated one's face is and the more one makes repeated facial movements over prolonged periods of time, the more the skin will show deepening wrinkles and furrows where the plane of the skin creases because of these movements. Therefore, this kind of indiscriminate exercising may hasten the development of facial lines and furrows. However, isometric exercises designed to ensure facial muscle balance have been found to be helpful. These exercises are useful in eliminating certain brow and forehead lines. We have described them on page 132 (Brow and Forehead Surgery).

Will face-lift surgery eliminate all my lines and make my face lose its character?

No. A face-lift will reduce the depth of certain lines or furrows and will generally make you look younger and more refreshed. It will not totally eliminate lines, grooves or furrows, and will not detract from the character your face possesses.

Am I neurotic for wanting a face-lift?

There is nothing neurotic about wanting to look your best. Many people remain very handsome as they age, but inevitably the combined results of prolonged exposure to sun, wind, other elements, emotions, dietary indiscretions and other things take their toll. Wishing to have your looks restored so you look younger and more refreshed may bring good feelings, provided you have realistic expectations of surgery.

Is acupuncture a reasonable method of getting my face lifted?

In general, Western medicine remains skeptical about acupuncture, although there seems to be evidence of its usefulness in certain situations. To date, there is no evidence we know of that acupuncture is useful for the kind of cosmetic repair accomplished by a face-lift.

I've noticed that my friend's wrinkles are different from mine. They seem finer, while my skin sags more. Can you explain these differences?

The quality of skin varies from person to person. Thicker, oilier skin ages with folds and becomes sagged, while thinner skin ages with parchment-like shallow creasing and fine wrinkles. Men's and women's skin age at different rates. Male skin appears thicker, reinforced by the hair follicles of the beard. These hair follicles do for the male complexion what steel mesh does for concrete—they provide built-in reinforcement.

What percentage of those requesting face-lifts are men?

More men are requesting face-lifts today than ever before. This may be due to greater acceptance of cosmetic surgery in general, or to increased male awareness of aging and cosmetic problems. At present, about 25 percent of my patients requesting a face-lift are men.

How long after a face-lift may I shave?

You may shave lightly about three days after the operation. You may shave with normal pressure about one week after surgery. You may notice that hair growth in the lifted areas may be slower than usual in the early healing phase.

I'm 55 and considering a face-lift operation. What medical condition would make me a high-risk candidate for this operation?

Your surgeon should take a complete medical history, and you must have a thorough examination with laboratory tests before any surgery can be done. Certain medical conditions will make you a high-risk candidate for surgery. They are:

—An uncontrolled heart condition or an irregular heart beat.
—Very high blood pressure.
—Any disease that causes bleeding or bruising easily or excessively.
—Any severe medical condition such as uncontrolled diabetes or kidney disease.
—Any severe anemia.
—Certain medications you may take for a medical condition, such as anticoagulants or steroids.

These various conditions do not necessarily preclude surgery, providing you are under good medical care and your condition is well controlled. Each case must be considered individually before a decision about surgery can be made.

I'm 45 years old. I've been a widow for two years. All the men I now meet are interested in younger women. I don't want to get involved with a much older man. Will a face-lift subtract years and be a good idea for me at this stage of life?

There is no doubt that a face-lift, if properly done, will subtract years from your face. The crux of this question is whether surgery is a good idea at this stage of your life. You may benefit greatly from a face-lift if you have come to terms with the loss of your husband. Bereavement varies from person to person.

If you have come to terms with your loss, and hope that by looking younger you may be more attractive to men your own age, your plan may be realistic. But entertain no illusions about it: a face-lift can make you look younger, but it will not change your personality and it is not a prescription for unbridled happiness. It is perfectly understandable that at this stage you may wish to begin anew. The good feelings you derive from your new look may make some important differences in how you perceive yourself and, therefore, in how others see you.

My husband has been dead for five years. I am 60 years old. He left me comfortable, and I am now considering a face-lift to make me more attractive. I feel guilty about spending his money so that I'll be able to meet someone to take his place. Are these feelings normal? Do I need help?

This is not unusual. People often feel guilty about many things after the death of a loved one. This is part of normal mourning. Mourning is an intense psychological process whose purpose is to relinquish the attachment to a loved one so that new attachments may be formed. This often involves guilty feelings. This is especially true weeks or months after a loved one's death. Some people may feel guilty about feeling good or even about laughing at a joke when a loved one has died a short while earlier.

There would be something wrong if such doubts and guilty feelings did not accompany your wishes to look younger and more attractive and perhaps eventually to meet someone else. But re-member, no future relationship or situation diminishes the life you and your husband had together.

I'm 38, married, and have a part-time job. My husband and I are not as sexually active as we were ten years ago and I'm afraid that I'm less attractive to him. He says there is nothing wrong. But I'm sure we would be more intimate if I looked the way I did when we first met. I think his lack of interest is because I'm starting to look middle-aged. Should I consider a face-lift?

Many married couples have an active sexual life well into their fifties, sixties and beyond. At 38, unless there is a very special cosmetic problem, you are on the young side for a face-lift. There can be many reasons a couple may be sexually less active than before and it is rare that such decreasing attraction has to do with either partner's growing older.

More likely, you and your husband have other difficulties that are affecting your intimate life. You should consider counseling together as a couple. One thing is certain. If your husband has lost interest, your having a face-lift will not rekindle the fire. You must explore the psychological problem, rather than try to alter super-ficial things.

Is there a best time of year for a face-lift?

There is no best time of the year for a face-lift. The major consideration is that you can take time to rest and recuperate. If you have specific allergies which act up in summer, then have the surgery at another time. You must also consider the sun. Can you refrain from excessive exposure? If sunbathing is important to you, you could have the surgery in late September, when the sunbathing season is over. That way you won't feel deprived over the next five or six months.

Can a face-lift correct my double chin?

By surgically removing the accumulation of fat beneath your skin, a face-lift can correct this condition. When you have your consultation, the surgeon should point out the specific cosmetic flaws detracting from your appearance. There should be a full discussion of these problems and of the procedures the surgeon will employ to correct them.

I've been told that a face-lift can give you a masklike, unnatural-looking face. Is that true?

A properly done face-lift will not give you a masklike, unnatural look. Instead, it will remove major folds, wrinkles and excess skin. For a few days after the procedure, the face may appear slightly swollen and smoothed out because of the swelling of the tissues after surgery. This is completely normal, and many patients report a taut sensation about the face and neck. This quickly subsides as the tissues become less swollen over the next two or three days. Some patients even express mild dissatisfaction as a few minor, fine wrinkles reappear on the face.

I'm a 32-year-old tennis pro at a resort. I'm disturbed by the crow's-feet that are now deepening around my eyes. They look even more conspicuous when I get a tan because they then look like white streaks. Will surgery correct this?

It is very difficult to eliminate crow's-feet lines. They are generally the beginning signs of the aging face. They are the normal result of having an animated face or of excessive squinting (being out in bright sunlight, etc.). These lines can be somewhat lessened by a face-lift, especially one that concentrates on the area of the temples. Chemical peeling is another method that may be used with some effectiveness. You would be well off to take measures against the sun so you will not squint so much. Squinting deepens the lines and prevents the sun from tanning that area, resulting in whitish lines radiating out from the corners of the eyes.

I'm a 55-year-old woman. It's been a year now since my face-lift and blepharoplasty. I was very satisfied with my results at first, but I'm having doubts now because nobody has commented that I look better.

Many patients who have had successful face-lift surgery make similar comments. They are often surprised that their friends and relatives don't comment more often on their new looks. There can be a number of reasons for this. First, someone may be embarrassed to mention anything if you look dramatically different. However, people who have had good surgical results should not look too dramatically different after their recovery period. The object of a face-lift is to make you look younger and more refreshed; you wouldn't want an appearance that would scream *face-lift!* You may hear some casual remarks about your looking refreshed or healthy, or perhaps a friend will suddenly comment that you've lost some weight. But generally, most patients hear very little from others about their successful surgery. Besides, it is unlikely anyone else was as tuned in to your preoperative looks as you yourself were. After all, no one scrutinizes your face as carefully as you yourself do. Also, one year later most people will have forgotten your preoperative looks. Consequently, it doesn't occur to them to comment on your new look, since it is now your usual look, which is quickly assimilated.

I'm a 50-year-old woman. I've been a little down in the dumps for the last five or six months. A friend recommended that I see a plastic surgeon about having a face-lift. She says that it could really "pick me up." Should I do this?

If you've been feeling blue there must be a reason for it. If your looks are getting you down, then surgery may be fine. But you must carefully assess your feelings. Something is getting you down enough for your friend to notice, or perhaps you've been upset enough to mention it to her. If there is an emotional problem, it's more important to deal with it than to have a face-lift. Has something happened within the last five or six months? Is there a change going on in your life? Has your youngest child moved out of the house? Has your husband been spending more time away from home? There may be many questions that need answering before you understand why you've been feeling down. You may wish to consider a consultation with a competent professional trained in dealing with emotional difficulties.

I'm going to have a face-lift in a few months. I live alone. Which is the best kind of facility for my postoperative recovery period?

You should discuss this important question with your surgeon. There are many options today. If your surgery is being done at a hospital, you may choose to spend the first three or four postoperative days there. If you will have surgery at an out-patient facility, arrangements can be made to accommodate you for the first few postoperative days. There are also special spas and health facilities specializing in postoperative care where you will be under the supervision of a directing physician. The important thing to remember is that it would be best to have someone with you during your first few postoperative days.

I live in a medium-sized midwestern city. I've heard that the best plastic surgeons are located in New York and California. Should I try finding a surgeon in those areas or should I consult with a board-certified plastic surgeon in my area?

No geographic area has a monopoly on surgical or medical expertise. There are many fine plastic surgeons located throughout the country. As mentioned in Chapter 1 ("Finding the Proper Surgeon"), many factors must be considered when deciding on a surgeon's credentials. Among them are the surgeon's experience, the volume of cosmetic surgery the physician does, and the rapport you can develop with the surgeon. You may obtain a list of qualified plastic surgeons in your area by writing or telephoning the American Society of Plastic and Reconstructive Surgeons at 29 E. Madison Street, Chicago, Illinois 60602. Chapter 2 provides a step-by-step approach to choosing a surgeon who will meet your needs.

EIGHT

Brow and Forehead Surgery

Lines and That Sleepy Look

With age, with the ever-present pull of gravity, and with excessive animation of the facial muscles, the forehead eventually becomes lined. Many people dislike these lines and want them removed or reduced in depth. Such lines are not necessarily the result of aging, although time certainly contributes to their formation. They can be caused by having a very animated face and by certain muscle imbalances, which we will discuss in another section of this chapter. The lines of the forehead are of two types: horizontal lines and vertical lines, often called "scowl" or "frown" lines, which form between the eyebrows and above the nose.

The other major effect of aging in this area is that of drooping eyebrows. This may occur at the outer (lateral) region of the brow, closer to the temple. It affects the most frequently observed area of your face—your eyes. If the drooping becomes severe, the entire cast of your face may change. We have already discussed (Chapter 6, Eyelid Surgery) how removal of excess skin from the upper and lower eyelids improves appearance. Part of the problem in the upper eyelid area is that excess skin can give the face a tired look. The eyes appear less wide open, less alert, and they take on a sleepy look. As described in Chapter 6, a blepharoplasty operation can return a crisp, alert look to the upper eyelids.

129

However, drooping of the *eyebrows* can add to the puffy appearance of the upper eyelid region. Failure to recognize this sometimes leads a patient to have an unnecessary blepharoplasty operation. This remedies the eyelid region, but doesn't correct the drooping *eyebrow*, which may be a major contributor to the problem. When a patient has a blepharoplasty but there is an uncorrected drooping eyebrow, the patient is plagued by the same problem that led to the surgeon's office in the first place!

If the eyebrows continue to droop, the tired look may progress to a scowling appearance, as though the person were always angry. This is usually caused by the development of deep vertical lines between the eyebrows.

To understand this common cosmetic problem it is helpful to discuss the anatomy of this area of the face.

Several muscles in this area work in opposition to each other. The *frontalis* muscle is located in the forehead and lifts the eyebrows, as when we look surprised. When this muscle contracts it causes the horizontal lines of the forehead to appear.

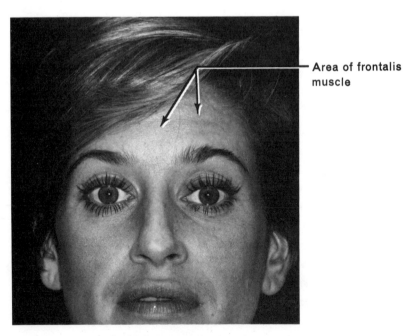

Area of frontalis muscle

The look of surprise.

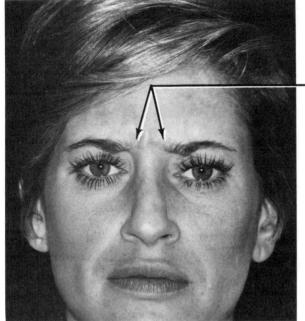

Area of corrugator
muscle

Scowling.

Opposing the frontalis muscle is a pair of muscles working to pull the eyebrows down into a scowl. These are the *corrugator* muscles, located at the sides of the nose in the eyebrow region. When they contract they oppose the frontalis, lowering the eyebrows and forming the vertical lines between the eyes.

Certain habits and external influences also can cause this effect. You should know about them because they may hasten and deepen the formation of these unattractive frown lines.

• Excessive squinting involves overusing the corrugator muscles to pull the eyebrows down, and may hasten and deepen scowl lines. Exposure to excessive sunlight without sunglasses may cause too much squinting. Frequent squinting also occurs in people with uncorrected vision problems, or in those who have light-sensitive eye conditions and don't wear sunglasses. Any vision or light-sensitive conditions you may have should be diagnosed and treated. This will lessen the need for squinting and reduce the use of the corrugator muscles.

• Excessive animation of the face may cause deepening of folds and wrinkles in all facial areas. The brow area is no exception. We all know people whose faces "light up" with laughter or other feelings. These are people whose emotions are readily expressed. Such people, though often ebullient and the center of attention, may pay a price for this in the changes that occur in their facial tissues. The character lines often seen on the faces of seasoned actors and actresses attest to this result of prolonged and frequent use of the facial muscles.

• Gravity also works to pull down the eyebrows.

There may be an *imbalance* in these opposing muscles, the frontalis and the corrugator muscles. This imbalance can cause the falling or drooping of the eyebrows and can result in a deepening of the vertical frown lines between the eyes. While surgery works to correct this imbalance, you must learn about the underlying cause of these furrows. Any existing muscle imbalance favors the corrugator muscles (because they have gravity on their side) and will eventually cause deepening of the scowl furrows.

Some people develop the habit of using their corrugator muscles excessively. They may be unaware that they are squinting or scowling even as they go about their daily routines. Sometimes, simply becoming aware that you are doing this helps you reduce or eliminate this scowling and squinting.

Your plastic surgeon may recommend a series of isometric exercises that are very effective in eliminating this scowling habit. This involves placing your palm across your forehead and then flexing the frontalis muscle as hard as you can by trying to raise your eyebrows against the downward pressure of your palm. This eventually strengthens the frontalis muscle, which must oppose the downward pull of the corrugators. After some weeks of regular exercises, the preexisting muscle imbalance may be lessened or even eliminated.

Some people have their frown lines surgically removed but end up undoing their surgical results by continuing to overuse the corrugator muscles after the operation. Unless the underlying cause (the muscle imbalance and the overuse of the corrugator muscles) is reduced or eliminated, you may have surgery only to notice that, over time, the brow begins to fall again, and the furrows deepen.

Surgical Corrections

There are various surgical procedures that can be used to correct these conditions. The choice of which procedure to use depends on the extent of the cosmetic problem, on the specific type of problem involved, and on what the patient and surgeon agree should be done to improve the patient's looks.

Treatment to Reduce Lines and Grooves of the Forehead

The earliest problems one may have are lines and grooves of the forehead that are visible even when you don't scowl or raise your eyebrows. The corrections for these cosmetic flaws are described in Chapter 9 (Chemical Peeling and Dermabrasion) and in Chapter 10 (Collagen Treatments).

Surgery to Correct Slight Drooping of the Eyebrow, Done Along With a Blepharoplasty

This procedure is an accompaniment to a blepharoplasty. It is done when a patient has slightly drooping eyebrows that contribute to the fullness of the upper eyelid and to the tired look. The correction can be done through the incision in the upper eyelid region, as part of the blepharoplasty. The brow is elevated by placing several sutures through the deeper layers of the skin beneath the eyebrow region, and attaching this to its former position higher up on the brow. This corrects the minor deformity of the drooping brow.

Surgery to Raise Drooping Eyebrows Without Blepharoplasty

Some patients require the raising of their drooping eyebrows alone, without an accompanying blepharoplasty. To raise the eye-

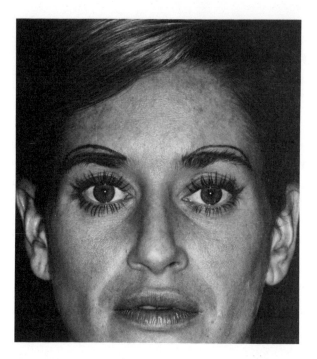

The direct approach for brow-lift. The markings demonstrate where the ellipse of skin will be removed. When the skin edges are sutured together the eyebrow is returned to its former higher position. The scar is camouflaged by the eyebrow itself.

brows and return them to their former position, several surgical approaches may be used.

First is a *direct* approach. This is done by making an incision at the top border of the eyebrow. An ellipse of skin is then removed and, when sutured, the eyebrow is returned to its higher, former position. The shape of the piece of skin to be removed is fashioned to allow for the appropriate correction. This procedure may be done in the doctor's office under local anesthesia.

A second method of raising the eyebrows is through an incision placed in the *hairline of the scalp*. This is done in the temple area.

Here, skin is removed, raising the tissues between the incision

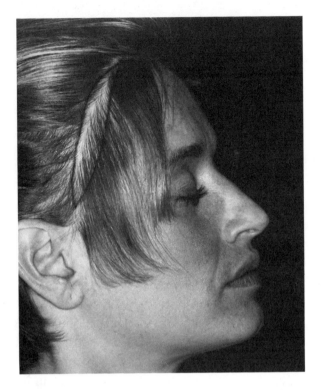

Scalp region approach for brow-lift. The markings
show the hidden position of the scar and the ellipse
of skin to be removed.

and the eyebrow. The ellipse of skin removed is adjusted to move
the eyebrow in the desired direction. The incision is well concealed
within the hair of the scalp. This procedure may also be done in
the surgeon's office under local anesthesia.

Raising the Eyebrows and Weakening the Corrugator Muscles

While procedures for restoring the proper position of the eyebrows can be very effective, they may not work well if the corrugator muscles are overactive. To maintain proper eyebrow position
in such cases, these corrugators may require weakening. Removal
of a segment of these muscles can be done directly through an

incision near the eyebrow, since the corrugator muscle lies immediately below the brow, near the nose. A significant portion of the muscle may be removed if necessary. It is very difficult to immobilize the corrugator muscle completely. Weakening the corrugators can make the restoration of a more youthful brow last much longer.

Raising the Eyebrows, Weakening the Corrugator and the Frontalis Muscles

Some patients may need the eyebrows raised and the corrugator muscles and the frontalis muscle weakened. This may be done when there are very deep horizontal lines across the forehead (caused by overuse of the frontalis muscle); when there are deep, vertical scowl lines (caused by overuse of the corrugator muscles); and when there is also great drooping of the eyebrows. The surgical approach is usually a coronal incision across the top of the head. Thus the surgeon has access to all muscles of the forehead region and can also elevate the eyebrows. The brow can be adjusted to allow elevation near the nose or at the lateral area on the side that most often droops.

In this procedure, the incision is made in the scalp and runs across the top of the head, usually at ear level. It is not necessary to shave the head. The skin is flapped downward to the eyebrow region. This allows the surgeon to reach the corrugator muscles, which can be weakened. The frontalis muscle can also be weakened. As the incision is closed, excess scalp is removed and the eyebrows are then set at the proper position. This procedure can be done in the surgeon's office under mild sedation and with local anesthesia.

All these procedures may be done independently of each other, depending on your specific cosmetic problem. They may also be combined either with eyelid surgery or with face-lift surgery, depending on the extent of the problem and on what you prefer to have done.

Frequently Asked Questions

Is there any danger that my brow won't be able to move after the muscles are weakened by forehead surgery?

No. After weakening the frontalis muscle or the corrugator muscles, there is movement left, regardless of how much of the muscle has been removed. It is difficult to immobilize these muscles permanently.

What are the complications that may attend this surgery?

As with almost any operation, the most likely complication has to do with the possibility of infection. In surgery of the face, head and neck, however, this complication is not frequent.

Excessive bleeding may be another complication. However, bleeding is scrupulously attended to during surgery. In surgery of the eyebrow region there may be black-and-blue areas after the operation. This rapidly dissipates over the next few days.

You may experience numbness if your surgeon uses a coronal incision when weakening the frontalis muscle and the corrugators. This may occur because some nerve endings in the incision area have been disturbed. With these approaches there is always the possibility that nerves traveling to the brow and hairline may be affected. This may produce numbness.

If I have a brow-lift, how long will my eyebrows stay up? Will they droop again in time?

This depends on the extent to which certain bad habits (squinting, scowling, etc.) and overuse of the muscles contribute to the problem. If you scrupulously practice your isometric exercises (see text on page 132) so as to offset any possible muscle imbalance, even with severe animation of your face the chances are good that your results will be long-lasting.

Can exercising my eyebrows return them to their normal position?

No. If overuse and overactivity of the muscles contribute to the problem, the tissues are already stretched and the eyebrows will droop. The exercises can be helpful to prevent further drooping after you have the problem corrected surgically. The exercises will prevent a quick reappearance of the scowl lines and drooping.

I know that local anesthesia numbs the area during surgery, but what about when I get home? Will I have pain?

There is surprisingly little, if any, pain after the operation in brow and forehead procedures. There may be some discomfort, which can be relieved by a mild analgesic. However, though aspirin is a fine analgesic, you must not use it postoperatively because it adds to the tendency to bleed. Use other compounds as prescribed by your physician.

How long will it be after brow surgery before I can return to work?

This depends on the extent of surgery you are having done. Many of these operations can be done before a weekend, and you may return to work on Monday with little or no discomfort or discoloration.

NINE

Chemical Peeling
and Dermabrasion

The face is the only area of the body where muscles attach directly to the deeper layers of the skin. With constant use and stretching, the skin eventually loses its tone, and wrinkles and lines appear. The skin is directly attached to the underlying muscles in the forehead region between the eyebrows, around the eyes and the mouth, and in the areas at the side of the nose leading to the mouth. After years of using these muscles, deep lines and grooves form in these areas. Although the rest of the facial skin may not have direct contact with the muscles, wrinkles may form in these areas as well, because of the stress from the adjacent areas. The lines in these nearby areas are not as deep as those formed by muscle contact; rather, they are caused by aging and by the ever-present pull of gravity. The skin reflects both its own aging process and the muscle activity beneath.

We have already discussed face- and brow-lifting, which are designed to remove excess stretched skin and to deal with underlying muscle problems. After these procedures, however, the remaining skin may still have some lines and wrinkles. When this is the case, chemosurgery (chemical peeling) and dermabrasion can be an enormous help. Also, in a younger person who is not yet ready for a face-lift, but where fine lines and wrinkles have appeared, these procedures can be very helpful. In these patients, the fine lines about the eyes or grooves in the upper lip into which cosmetics may run can be a great source of annoyance.

For older patients, these techniques may be used in conjunction with face- and brow-lift procedures to remove any remaining fine lines not eliminated by the surgery.

Both chemical peeling and dermabrasion remove superficial layers of the skin, allowing for growth of a new outer layer, which appears smoother and free of wrinkles. The procedures of chemical peeling and dermabrasion (along with collagen treatments, to be discussed in the next chapter) may be blended into an overall plan for facial rejuvenation. Since there are important differences between chemical peeling and dermabrasion, we will describe them separately.

Chemical Peeling

This process (also referred to as chemosurgery) is the application of a caustic material to remove the upper layers of the skin. This is effective for removing fine lines, irregular pigmentation, and some other imperfections of the skin. After removal of the upper layers, a crust forms and a new layer of skin forms beneath the crust. Chemical peeling can be used in the areas of the eyelids and the hairline, where dermabrasion cannot be used. It is also used in areas about the mouth and for fine wrinkles over all areas of the face.

When used in conjunction with face-lift surgery, the area of treatment is confined to the region of the lips. No areas directly undergoing surgery should be treated with the chemical solution. Of course, since face-lifting will reduce many lines of the face, chemosurgery is usually used after the face-lift to remove any remaining lines. It is another method of fine-tuning following a face-lift.

Before Having Chemical Peeling

It is especially important before chemosurgery to have a full medical examination, since the caustic agent most often used is a chemical called phenol. When phenol is used (even on the skin), some of this chemical is absorbed into the body. The liver and kidneys act on the absorbed phenol to eliminate it. Therefore, any patient with a history of liver or kidney problems should be scrupulously evaluated before chemical peeling. Also, since irregular heartbeats may occur because of the absorption of small amounts of phenol through the skin, any history of heart problems —no matter how minor—must be brought to your surgeon's attention.

The following are some other items of information you need to know before undergoing chemosurgery:

> The nature of your skin is an important consideration when deciding if you are an appropriate candidate for this treatment. Thin-skinned, blond, light-complexioned people are the best candidates for chemosurgery. With people whose skin is darker, blotching and discoloration of the treated area becomes an increasing possibility.
>
> Chemosurgery is usually limited to the face region. Treatments applied to the neck area have a much higher incidence of scarring.
>
> Beauty marks (technically called nevi) may become darker after chemosurgery. This is because of the loss of the superficial layers of skin over their pigments. Also, pore size may become enlarged in the treated area after chemosurgery.

When careful consideration is given to these important factors and limitations, chemical peeling is a safe and effective method for rejuvenating the face. You should discuss all these factors with your surgeon before beginning any such chemosurgery.

How Chemosurgery Is Done

Chemosurgery may be done in your doctor's office or in a hospital. Your skin is prepared with an antiseptic soap and thoroughly cleansed. Ether is then applied. This eliminates the oil normally present in skin, allowing a more complete application of the solution and better adherence of the surgical tape.

The phenol solution is applied with cotton applicators. As it is swabbed on your skin, you may feel a mild burning sensation. Some patients report a tingling feeling. This is not painful, since the phenol itself is a local anesthetic. The area of application is gently swabbed, and the solution is feathered and applied in decreasing amounts toward the periphery of the treatment site. The solution is applied in a slow, deliberate manner to minimize the amount of phenol absorbed through the skin.

The solution is confined to facial skin only. Facial skin is rich in blood supply, hair follicles and sebaceous glands. This means that facial skin can regenerate more quickly than skin elsewhere, once the caustic solution has been applied.

Your surgeon may decide to allow the chemical to work more deeply. This is done by applying a waterproof adhesive tape over the treatment area. This is known as an occlusive dressing. The adhesive tape prolongs the action of the chemical and allows it to penetrate deeper into the skin layers. With this technique, your surgeon can adjust the chemical treatment to the characteristics of your skin.

The tape mask is held in place for 24 to 48 hours. During this time you must remain fairly stationary and should refrain from talking unnecessarily. This is to prevent disturbing the tape-mask and the underlying tissue. Liquids may be taken through a straw if the area near the mouth has been treated and masked. Pain medications (such as Tylenol or aspirin) may be taken if necessary.

The swelling of the treated skin may become more noticeable by 48 hours as some clear fluid weeps from beneath the mask. At 48 hours you must return to the surgeon's office for removal of the adhesive mask. If limited areas of the face have been treated, this is not painful. If larger areas have been treated, analgesics may be necessary. After the tape is removed, the skin is red, moist and swollen. The treated area is dusted with an antiseptic powder, which adheres to the surface. A crust forms over the treated area.

You will be instructed to apply the antiseptic powder until the crust dries. An ointment is then applied to the crusted surface. This softens it, so that it will easily separate from the underlying new skin. Depending on the depth of the treatment, the crust soon separates and falls away. At that point you may gently wash your face with ordinary soap and water. You must not pick at any remaining crust. Some physicians prescribe a steroid ointment to be applied to the area. Steroids, with their anti-inflammatory action, reduce the redness and swelling of the treated area.

As early as 10 to 14 days after treatment, hypoallergenic makeup (makeup with components which are less likely to cause allergic or irritative reactions) may be used for short periods of time each day. Your new skin layer is pink and smooth, and feels very tight. Most patients are excited and happy when they see this new layer of skin. Although it feels taut and is pink (the color will eventually fade), they are delighted at the wrinkle-free condition of their faces.

After Chemosurgery

The skin appears pink in most cases. This color may remain for 8 to 12 weeks, although during that time you can cover the affected area with makeup. In time this discoloration will subside. Your skin will be smoother and have far fewer wrinkles around the mouth, on the cheeks, and at the corners of the eyes.

There is one major precaution you must know about: You must not expose your face to the sun for six months after chemosurgery. The skin is highly sensitive to the sun's ultraviolet rays; most cases of blotchy pigmentation after chemosurgery are caused by early exposure to the sun. In tropical climates you must be especially careful, since even reflected sun can cause a problem. There are specific blocking agents to protect your skin from the sun.

Possible Complications

Though chemosurgery is safe when done by properly trained practitioners, there may be complications. They are:

The treated skin may become lighter than the surrounding untreated area. If the transition from light to dark skin is abrupt and therefore noticeable, a second chemical peel without occlusive tape may solve the problem. Makeup, of course, can also be helpful.

Increased color (known as hyperpigmentation) may occur in the treated area. This is more prone to happen in dark-skinned people and especially if the patient is exposed to direct sun too soon after chemosurgery. It may leave a blotchy appearance. The area of discoloration should fade within some weeks. If it does not, it can be treated by having another chemical peel some time later when the treated area has fully healed.

Occasionally scarring may occur if the solution penetrates too deeply or if areas other than the face (for instance, the neck) are treated. This is minimized by skillful application of the solution so that it does not penetrate too deeply and cause any burning of the deeper layers of skin.

There is another beneficial effect of chemical peeling you should be aware of. Besides having fewer wrinkles, the treated skin maintains certain qualities seen in younger skin. Some researchers have noted that microscopic examination shows the skin takes on certain characteristics associated with younger skin.

Frequently Asked Questions

I've been told that a beautician can do chemical peeling; that I don't have to go to a physician. Is this true?

Chemical peeling must be done by skilled and experienced practitioners. Chemosurgery, if improperly done, can lead to serious cases of scarring, burning, and even toxic reactions to the phenol used in the solution. These possible complications make it wiser to have chemosurgery done by an experienced physician. Before such surgery is done, a thorough medical history must be taken. It may be necessary to combine this with a physical examination and with pertinent laboratory tests to ensure that your kidneys and liver are functioning properly. Close medical scrutiny may be required during the procedure to preclude any difficulties. These safeguards can be assured if a properly trained physician performs this procedure.

Will chemical peeling remove the deep lines and creases on my face?

Chemical peeling is not a substitute for or an alternative to a face-lift operation. It is used to remove *fine wrinkling* only. Deep folds and creases are only slightly affected by chemosurgery. Such cosmetic problems require the techniques discussed in the chapters concerning face-lift, brow-lift and collagen treatments.

May I have chemical peeling after I've had a face-lift?

This is frequently done for patients who have both deep folds and creases, *and* the fine wrinkles that can be eliminated by chemosurgery. Some time after the face-lift, the chemical peel is performed. In a sense, the chemosurgery fine-tunes the face-lift.

I live in Florida. Can I safely have a chemical peel?

In the semitropical climate of Florida, the sun's ultraviolet rays are intense, even if you are not in direct sunlight. When out-of-doors you must take the proper precautions. Wear a wide-brimmed hat and cover the treated area with a total sunblock containing para-amino benzoic acid (P.A.B.A.) and zinc oxide or titanium dioxide. With these precautions many patients have had excellent results. Some of the leading clinical investigations of chemical peeling have been done with patients living in Florida.

My face was lifted and looks great! But my hands and arms give me away. Can they be peeled?

Chemosurgery should be done on *facial skin only!* Skin on the rest of the body, if treated by this method, may scar severely. There are other medications to help in the areas of the backs of the hands and the forearms. They act to remove the areas of pigmentation (sometimes known as age spots) and help to give a younger look to this skin.

How much does chemabrasion cost?

This, of course, depends on the size of the area to be treated. A full-face chemabrasion costs between $1,500 to $2,500.

I've heard that chemabrasion can be performed at the same time as a face-life. Is this true?

Yes, it can. However, there are limiting factors. Chemabrasion should only be performed on areas not being "lifted" directly. This limits the area of treatment to the skin of the upper and lower lip region. One must also remember that with chemabrasion there will be increased swelling after the operation. As with any well-designed surgical plan, your specific requirements and in-depth discussion with your surgeon will ensure the best arrangement for you.

Dermabrasion

This process involves the mechanical removal of the superficial layers of the skin. While similar to chemical peeling, it lends itself better to the treatment of acne and other depressed scars of facial skin. It is also useful for people for whom phenol cannot be used because they have some impairment of the liver or kidneys.

In this procedure, a high-speed, rotating steel brush, or some other abrasive material, is used to "sand down" the skin. It can effectively reduce minor hills and valleys caused by scar tissue, blending them into the surrounding skin.

The procedure requires anesthesia. The type of anesthesia used depends on the extent of the area to be treated. Usually, small areas of facial skin are treated, and the dermabrasion may be done under local or topical anesthesia. Topical sprays are used by some physicians. They not only anesthetize the skin but momentarily freeze it. This can be a great advantage, because the high-speed steel brush abrades the superficial skin layers more easily while they are firm.

The technique tapers the area of treatment to allow for a smooth transition from the deeply treated central area of the site to the lightly treated periphery adjacent to the untreated surrounding skin. This effect can be achieved by applying greater pressure and longer time of dermabrasion over the center of the treatment site and by applying less pressure for a shorter time toward the periphery of the area.

After the treatment, a crust develops over the treated area. At about the fifth to seventh day, the patient begins to apply a generous layer of ointment, which helps separate the crust. The patient is instructed not to remove the crust forcibly but to allow it to separate on its own. When it separates, it reveals a new, pink layer of skin.

After Dermabrasion

With dermabrasion, as with chemosurgery, the pink color of the skin lasts for about 12 weeks. You must avoid sunlight during the first six months after dermabrasion and should venture into the sun only with the proper protection.

The possible complications with this procedure are the same as those with chemosurgery, except for the possible danger involved with phenol. They are:

Hyperpigmentation. This appears to be related to exposure to the sun too soon after having undergone dermabrasion.

Minor scarring. This is infrequent.

Frequently Asked Questions

I have dark skin, brown eyes and brown hair. Am I a good candidate for dermabrasion?

As with chemosurgery, the best candidates for dermabrasion are people with fair skin. If you are darker-skinned, you run the risk of developing areas of darkened skin (hyperpigmentation). Such areas usually fade after a time. If they do not, they may be removed by additional chemosurgery. Your surgeon will discuss your specific skin color and any possible complications.

How long must I plan to be away from school if I'm going to have dermabrasion?

Allow about two weeks for recuperating after having dermabrasion. You should plan this procedure for a time when you have a vacation (for example, Christmas) or during the summer. If done during the summer, however, you must remember the precautions concerning the sun.

How much will dermabrasion cost?

As with chemabrasion, this will depend on the size of the area treated. The fees range up to $2,000.

I have lines in my upper lip. I have heard different opinions about which procedure is more suited to removing these lines. Which one should I choose—dermabrasion or chemabrasion?

Many factors should be evaluated to answer this question. For cosmetic improvement of fine lines in the upper and lower lip regions, the two methods can be equally effective. However, your age, general health, and type of skin will all come to bear on your surgeon's final decision.

TEN

Collagen Treatments

Surgery alone cannot eliminate all skin imperfections. Face- and brow-lift procedures work to eliminate deep folds and creases, but these cannot be totally erased. Some fine lines may still remain after surgery. In younger people, who are not yet candidates for face-lift surgery, the beginning furrows and fine lines may be very upsetting. These require some treatment by which they can be filled in or plumped up.

Liquid silicone was first used to fill such areas and lines in 1965. This material is injected beneath the skin and acts as a space-occupier. It is a liquid and remains in liquid form within the body. Because of this, silicone has been known to migrate to other locations in the body. In some cases, liquid silicone, after being injected into facial skin, has been found in the liver and kidneys. There is no evidence to date that this substance damages these organs. It sits inertly and does not interact chemically with the tissues. It is viewed by the body as foreign and, as such, is not incorporated into its tissues.

Liquid silicone is now being extensively studied by the FDA. It has never been approved for medical use by this agency. Although many physicians feel it is a worthwhile material for improving fine skin defects, there is no control over its manufacture and therefore over the purity of silicone used for these injections. You should be alerted to this and should question your physician about the source of any injectable liquid silicone to be used in your face.

In 1981 the FDA approved Zyderm™, a suspension of purified cattle collagen that comes in liquid form, for injection into facial skin. Collagen, a protein, is the structural building block of all essential body tissues, including skin. The concept behind collagen's use is that it fills up the depressed or deficient areas of facial skin with a latticework of purified collagen. In time, the patient's own blood vessels and cells move into the areas to occupy the structural scaffolding. This makes the injected implant a living part of the skin! It does not migrate. All evidence to date indicates that Zyderm is perfectly safe for injection into facial skin.

Before beginning collagen injection treatments, you must be skin-tested. A small number of people have had allergic reactions to Zyderm. Zyderm is not used on anyone with a personal or family history of an autoimmune disease (for example, arthritis or lupus erythematosis). The skin test is innocuous and is much like a t.b. test. A small amount of collagen is injected into the skin of the forearm and the area is then observed for one month for evidence of a local reaction.

Collagen does not work at certain sites and for certain kinds of depressed skin scars. It cannot be viewed as a replacement for a surgical face-lift. Furrows and grooves as well as fine lines of the skin are due not only to creasing and folding of the skin in the local area, but also to the falling of tissues as they weaken and stretch with age. Such defects may be remedied by face-lift surgery. Collagen injections are an excellent way of fine-tuning a face-lift after fallen tissues have been returned to their normal positions and excess skin has been removed by surgery.

The treatments themselves are nonsurgical and can be performed in the physician's office. No anesthesia or special preparation is required. The collagen is injected through a fine-gauge needle into the skin that is to be treated. Generally, two to six treatments spaced two weeks apart are needed to restore the area to a more youthful-looking appearance. Since collagen is in a

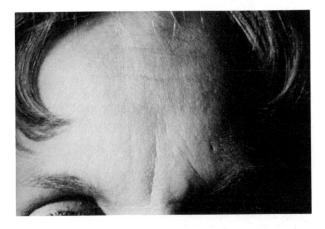

Frown line before Zyderm treatment.

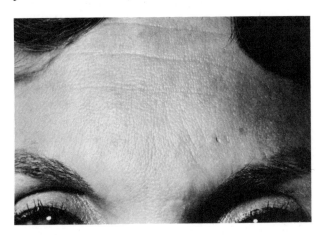

Frown line after Zyderm treatment.

solution that will be absorbed by the body, there will be an over-plump appearance of the treated area for a short time following the injection. Soon afterward, the area will recede to the level of the surrounding skin.

Long-term success with collagen is still being evaluated. At present there is some doubt about the permanence of the results. The product manufacturer suggests that touch-ups may be necessary after about two years.

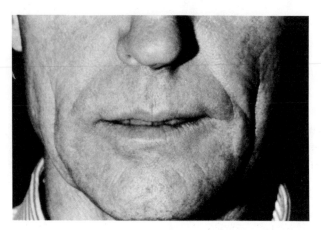

Age-related wrinkles before Zyderm treatment.

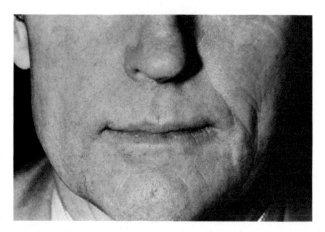

After Zyderm treatment.

At the time of this writing, a more concentrated form of injectable collagen has been placed on the market by the same manufacturer. The Zyderm company has been very active in the quality control of its product and in controlling its use. This kind of treatment is done only by physicians who have been given special training in the use of injectable collagen. In our opinion, the need for such a product seems great and the drawbacks and risks associated with collagen treatment seem minimal.

Frequently Asked Questions

If some M.D.'s claim that liquid silicone is good, why is it not available or at least tested?

As a safeguard to the public, any injectable material must pass the scrutiny of the FDA. This government agency maintains stringent standards for any drug or material that is to be used by the public. Silicone is still under investigation and has been since 1965. The latest study was scheduled to be made public in October 1981. At the time of this writing, the results are still pending. This study, unfortunately, does not contain conclusions about the use of liquid silicone for eliminating fine lines and wrinkles of the face. It concerns the use of liquid silicone for more serious tissue deficiencies. We can only hope that future research will shed more light on this important area.

I have forehead lines. Can they be treated by having collagen injections?

Yes, they can be treated effectively. However, with such lines we think it would be helpful for you to seek out their cause. Sometimes they are due to aging, which is beyond your control. Sometimes the falling of forehead and brow tissues adds to these lines. A complete evaluation should be made to determine if you can delay these lines from returning once they are improved or eliminated. As was mentioned in Chapter 8 (Brow-Lift), certain isometric exercises may be very beneficial in delaying the return of forehead lines once they have been eliminated or reduced in depth. In other instances, where the lines are due to aging and the falling of tissues, surgery may be the most appropriate treatment.

Is the liquid silicone used in facial injections the same as that used in chin and breast implants?

No. All silicone is made from the same basic chemical unit. But as more silicone molecules are chemically linked together, the substance becomes firmer. Liquid silicone remains liquid after being injected into the skin. The silicone used in chin and breast implants are not liquids. They are soft, solid materials. They remain solid once they are implanted within the chin or the breast area. They cannot migrate, as has occasionally happened with liquid silicone used in facial injections.

I have had liquid silicone injected into my face before. Does this mean I am going to have trouble because of this at some time in the future?

Not at all. Most patients receiving liquid silicone injections have had very gratifying results. Many physicians experienced with injectable silicone have suggested that knowing how to use, and where to inject, the material prevents it from migrating to other parts of the body. They claim that any past problems were caused by two things: Too much silicone was used, and the material was impure or was not medical-grade silicone.

In our opinion, the chances are that if you've had silicone injections with pleasing results you will remain pleased and there will be no future difficulty. To the best of our knowledge, there is no evidence that silicone that has migrated to other organs has caused any damage.

ELEVEN

Other Surgical Procedures

Many other cosmetic surgical procedures can be performed on the face and neck regions. In this chapter we will briefly discuss the most common ones so you will have an overview of the range of cosmetic facial operations being done today.

Surgery of the Ears

Protrusion of the ears is a fairly common cosmetic flaw. It is an inborn trait for some people, just as is the shape of the nose or chin. Protruding ears may be caused by overgrowth of the cup portion (or concha) of the ear, or it may be caused by failure of the ear parts to fold properly. Sometimes a combination of these factors causes the ear to protrude. If the ears protrude greatly, this detracts from a person's looks. Men and women alike are affected by this problem. If someone decides to have surgery to eliminate the protrusion, the specific ear part involved determines the type of operation necessary.

Unlike the rest of the face or body, the ears reach 85 percent of their final adult height by the time a child is four years old. This rapid growth means that protruding ears appear at a very early age. An eight- or ten-year-old child who, because of protruding ears, has been subjected to the comments of other children for the last five or six years may develop lasting feelings of unworthiness. These feelings may focus on the ears alone, or they may become part of the child's view of his or her entire self.

Young children who are ridiculed about their ears may not tell their parents about their feelings. Instead, they may come to view themselves as unworthy, and the emotional burden is then greater than if the child simply focused on the ear deformity.

Parents, of course, notice the deformity but may be reluctant to mention it. Or they may not want to impose their personal feelings on the child. They may ignore the issue until years later when the child, older and more verbal, expresses dissatisfaction with his or her looks. Meanwhile, years have passed and the child may have endured the comments and jokes of other children all this while.

As the child matures, the rest of the head and neck finally catch up to the ears in size. Thus the protruding ears may become less obvious, although they still stick out. But the psychological damage may already have been done and the person may still see himself or herself as having unsightly and protruding ears.

DORA L. was a 36-year-old woman who came to my office. "I want my ears pinned back," she said, stroking her longish hair, which completely covered her ears. She detailed how as a child she had been called names because of her large and protruding ears. When she was old enough to decide for herself, she chose hair styles that covered her ears. She had worn her hair long ever since that time. "I always felt I was hiding something," she said. "Like I had this ugly little secret which a boyfriend would eventually find out about. And *then* . . . what would I do?"

Despite this "deformity," as she termed it, she had a normal social life. With her marriage her concerns about her ears lessened and she felt much better about herself. But when the marriage dissolved, Dora's bad feelings about her ears surfaced once again. She began gazing at her ears in the mirror, something she hadn't done since her adolescence. Finally, at the age of 36, she decided to "do something about a problem that's plagued me all my life."

When I examined her ears, I was surprised to see that, although they protruded, they were not as large or unsightly as Dora L's description had led me to believe. Though as a child Dora's ears may have protruded in comparison to her other features, as time passed her ears had become more harmoniously balanced with the rest of her features, which had nearly caught up with her ears. However, her negative feelings about her ears remained.

While Dora L's ears did protrude, it was clear to me that she had an exaggerated view of their size and shape. She had retained an inner emotional view of herself that included *very large* and protruding ears. Realistically, she was a very attractive woman. But she wanted ear surgery. Her recent divorce with its emotional stress had reactivated the old feelings of worthlessness—feelings that focused on her ears and spread to her entire view of herself.

I attempted to help Dora reconcile her emotional concern about her "deformity," without success. Dora was not a good surgical candidate at this time. I recommended that she seek psychological counseling prior to any surgery.

Ear deformities may be repaired as early as four or five years of age. If the child is properly prepared for surgery, if he or she is told about it and trusts the parents and the surgeon, the surgery goes very well. Surgery at this early age will insure that the child never experiences ridicule from other children about the size of his or her ears. Of course, we are talking about a situation where there is a *true* ear deformity, and where the child will most likely have to endure years of comments from other children. Many adults, like Dora L., recall having tolerated taunts and name-calling for years, all the while carrying this physical and emotional burden. Only at a later point in their lives do they decide to have ear surgery.

With ear surgery, the procedure and method of anesthesia

used is determined by the type of problem and by the particular patient's needs and preferences. Children are usually operated on while under general anesthesia, while adults may choose to have local anesthesia and i.v. sedation.

The ears can be made to look completely normal with this surgery. An occasional postoperative patient may develop thickened scars located behind the ears, but this is barely visible.

There are other cosmetic ear problems that can be surgically corrected. Some people have ear lobes that are very long and droop. Other people may be dissatisfied because their ear lobes do not have the usual attachment to the side of the face. There may instead be a cleft between the skin of the lobe and the face. Although these cosmetic flaws are minor, they can sometimes be annoying and a source of concern. After all, we are talking about elective surgical procedures to make cosmetic corrections and to satisfy individual preferences. Some women are particularly sensitive to ear imperfections, since earrings call attention to the ears.

Various in-office procedures are performed under local anesthesia to correct these cosmetic problems. Your surgeon will use a surgical technique that is individually tailored to your specific cosmetic needs.

Aging may present ear problems, just as it does with other facial features. Some older people develop fine lines and wrinkles on their ear lobes. This may be quite distressing to someone who has had a face-lift with fine results, but who feels the ear lobes tell the truth. The same procedures used on certain other facial areas (for instance, chemical peeling) can be used to eliminate these lines and wrinkles.

After years of wearing heavy jewelry on their ears, some women find that their ear lobes elongate and droop. Ear-lobe tissue loses its elasticity with time, as does the tissue throughout the rest of the face and neck. Again, there are various in-office surgical procedures to correct these problems.

Pierced earrings may occasionally cause injury to the ear lobes. An earring may snag on clothing or be accidentally pulled, causing a tear in the delicate tissue of the lobe. For some people, years of wearing heavy earrings may cause enlargement of the hole in the lobe. These injuries can be repaired with excellent results. Usually, surgery is performed in an office setting. The repair can be done so that earrings may again be worn after the tissue of the ear lobe has completely healed.

Your surgeon will be glad to examine your ears and to make suggestions about any flaw you have that bothers you. The techniques used to correct these minor but annoying problems are individually tailored for the specific cosmetic problem you may have.

Adjustment of the Upper and Lower Lips

A patient may have a thick upper or lower lip, or both lips may be thick and full. These conditions can be surgically corrected. This involves the removal of excess lip tissue and the judicious placing of surgical incisions so there is minimal scarring. There are various flaws requiring different incisions and procedures. The incisions are not always in the mouth; sometimes the junction of the red portion of the lip and the surrounding skin is used. This area usually heals well, leaving an imperceptible scar.

The lip area is affected by the surrounding facial structures. For instance, the upper lip may be changed significantly with nasal surgery because the septum of the nose may pull the upper lip in an upward direction. Also, muscles of the lip are connected to the nose. The appearance of the nose and the lip together is important. Each facial structure is affected by its adjacent structures.

The lower lip is affected by the appearance of the chin beneath it. It can appear quite full and pouting when someone has a recessed or deficient chin. This may be brought into a more harmonious relationship when a chin implant is used. It is again important to realize that *facial harmony* is the major factor in determining overall good looks. With any intended surgery, especially affecting the lips, don't be surprised if your surgeon makes suggestions concerning other facial features. Remember, the more subtle the complaint, the more important is the interaction of your features to create an overall harmonious unity.

Correction of Facial Scars

Facial scars can be acquired through trauma or disease. No matter what its cause, a scar often reflects a wound in the psychological sense. Most people are concerned when they feel they have lost some aspect of their normal appearance. Many people who become scarred may begin to focus their attention on the scar and to feel that their general looks are affected. For some people, an unattractive scar makes them feel as though they *themselves* have become unattractive, both physically and as a person in the total sense of the word. The scar's presence may be an unpleasant reminder of the accident that caused the scar. Extensive scars (such as those from burns) can cause great psychological damage to someone's entire concept of the self and may radically change a person's life.

There are many types of scars, and there are various surgical techniques to deal with them cosmetically. Each patient's problem must be evaluated individually and then specifically treated. This can be done in an office visit. There are certain important principles you should know about scar corrections.

Most scars, no matter how unsightly, can be made to appear less noticeable with the proper surgical techniques. For example, a wide, jagged scar with discolored scar tissue can be revised so that it then becomes finer and straighter and will be less conspicuous than it was before the surgical procedure. This can greatly improve a patient's appearance.

There is no such thing as surgery or scar correction that leaves *absolutely no scar*. To expect such results would be unrealistic. While most scars can be improved or made to appear less conspicuous, some scar tissue will be left in place. The surgeon must meticulously plan the scar-correction operation, making allowances for many factors. These are: the patient's skin texture, the location of the scar, the elasticity of the skin, the direction of the underlying muscle layers, the width and depth of the scar, and the shape of the scar. There are other elements as well. These may include the patient's age, capacity to heal properly, and so on.

If you have an unsightly scar and are thinking of having a surgical correction, you and your surgeon should discuss the procedure. The surgeon will be able to tell you how he is planning your surgical correction. Various surgical techniques for scar correction are used in different situations. Techniques we have described in previous chapters may be used in addition to surgery. These include dermabrasion and collagen treatments.

You and your surgeon should discuss all the details of any intended scar-correction surgery. Doing this will keep you well informed so you will have reasonable and realistic expectations about the degree of cosmetic improvement you can hope to achieve.

Lasers and Cosmetic Facial Surgery

The word *laser* stands for Light Amplification by Stimulated Emission of Radiation. Its beam is an intense almost parallel beam of electromagnetic energy of a given wavelength or color. The type of laser determines the specific wavelengths it can produce. Certain tissues of the body will absorb certain wavelengths. The laser works by the transfer of the beam's light energy into heat energy. When this transfer occurs, the tissue absorbing the laser energy can be heated enough to vaporize, leaving a small nonbleeding border. The laser is a tool, as the scalpel is a tool, and is used by surgeons in many areas of the body. Lasers have been in use for approximately 25 years and are constantly being applied to new surgical tasks.

In the area of cosmetic facial surgery, the Argon laser in particular has been successful in the treatment of port wine stains. The port wine stain is a purple to blueish discoloration of the skin, frequently found in the face and neck area. Some work is also being done with the laser treatment of tattoos and other skin problems. At present lasers are not routinely used in any of the cosmetic surgical procedures presented here.

Frequently Asked Questions

My eight-year-old son's ears come to a point. He is teased and called "elf" and "Mr. Spock," after the character from Star Trek. *He enjoyed this at first, but now it's starting to concern him. Is there a surgical procedure to correct this problem?*

Yes, there is a relatively simple surgical procedure to correct this problem. The excess skin and cartilage of the ear can be removed, and the ear can be reshaped to produce a more normally shaped and attractive ear.

My five-year-old son has protruding ears. I want him to have surgery, especially now, since he will soon begin school. But my husband feels it would be taking an unnecessary risk. He says our son will "grow into" his ears and that the operation could be dangerous. Is he being overly cautious or am I too ready to take our son to a surgeon?

Your concerns are very understandable. Surgery should not be done unless there is a real cosmetic problem, one that will cause your son to endure ridicule and teasing at the hands of the other kids. Children can be quite cruel in their frankness, and this can cause a great deal of emotional pain. You should arrange for a consultation with a surgeon to determine if there is a significant cosmetic flaw that can or should be corrected by surgery. Your husband's concern is also understandable. While ear surgery is quite safe, surgery of any kind always carries some built-in risks. Rest assured, however, that ear surgery is performed routinely with good results. Be careful about expressing your doubts and concerns in your child's presence. After consulting with a plastic surgeon your fears and concerns should be eased. His confidence about any necessary surgery will be transmitted to your child.

Our son is four years old and will have his ears "pinned back" this summer. We don't want to frighten him but we want him to be aware of the procedure and prepared for any postoperative discomfort. How do we prepare a four-year-old child for cosmetic surgery?

This is an important question we believe every parent should be concerned about. It is very important that your child be told about his surgical experience beforehand. This will allow him time to ask questions and to feel more comfortable with the idea of surgery and a hospital setting. You don't want him forming incorrect ideas and fantasies about surgery. Also, you do not want him to think there is something fundamentally wrong with *him* as a person. At four years of age, a child has ideas about his body that do not conform to those of an adult. He is particularly prone to forming incorrect ideas about himself from misperceived impressions.

A child need not be told all the surgical details. It would be better to demonstrate to him by bending his ears gently back into the normal position so he can see exactly what the surgery will accomplish. There should be no mystery about it. Tell him there will be no pain or discomfort but that he will go to sleep for a short time during the operation. Tell him that when he awakes you will be there with him and that there will be bandages over his ears. Demonstrate what the bandages will be like. Keep your explanations simple, accurate and undetailed so that he may fully grasp the meaning of the situation.

My daughter is five and wears her hair tucked behind her ears. My mother says I shouldn't allow her to do this because the hair will force her ears forward and create a permanent protuberance of the ears. Is this right?

This is a myth. The cartilage of the ear is resilient, and your daughter's hair worn behind her ears will not cause them to change their shape or position.

My 18-month-old son sucks his thumb and folds his ear over with his other hand. I'm afraid this will give him deformed ears. Is this true?

The ear is composed of strong cartilage. This tissue will not be changed in shape or position by any manipulations your son is doing.

My ear lobes are so small that I can barely wear earrings. There isn't enough space to support more than the tiniest, lightest pair. Can my ear lobes be built up?

At the present time there is no operation to make a person's ears or ear lobes larger in size without scarring. Changes in size and shape can be made. Such reconstructive surgery is often done, for example, with trauma and burn patients. The tissue may have to be transferred from another part of the body. Frequently, the area behind the ear is a good source of tissue. This will leave some scarring behind the ears.

My lips appear crooked. One side of the bow of the upper lip is noticeably higher than the other. Is there a way to correct this?

Yes. This is not an uncommon cosmetic problem. It can be corrected by surgery. If your lips are a source of annoyance to you, you should consult with a plastic surgeon about having them re-shaped.

We are thinking of having our seven-year-old son's ears "pinned back" because he's been teased unmercifully at school. Is there any danger that this operation could impair his hearing?

Reshaping of the ears (called an otoplasty) is surgery done on the external ear only. The surgery has nothing to do with the ear canal or with the middle or inner ears, those parts of the ear concerned with hearing and equilibrium. The surgery will not harm your child's hearing. It is relatively uncomplicated surgery and is safe for both adults and children.

As an adult is it too late for me to have an otoplasty?

The surgical correction of protruding ears is not limited to children. We do recommend that this surgery be done as soon as is reasonably possible if a child has a serious cosmetic problem. But there is no age limit for this procedure. There are probably more adults than children having otoplasty each year.

After an otoplasty, will I have noticeable scars?

In surgery for protruding or overly large ears, the incisions are made behind the ears in the natural fold of the skin. The scars heal well and are not ordinarily visible to other people. There is no incision made in front of the ear during this procedure, and the scars do not present problems for patients.

How long after my ear operation will I be able to begin wearing my eyeglasses?

For about three to five days after surgery, you must wear a dressing over your ears. Glasses may be worn, if necessary, and held with tape outside the bandage. After removing the bandage, you may wear your glasses as usual. Your surgeon may suggest that you use a small gauze bandage for a few days longer, so that the eyeglass frame does not irritate the incision.

I have dark skin and have the tendency to form keloids. The keloid on my chin is very distressing and I would like to have this scar removed. But I've been told that if an incision is made into the scar, it will just form another keloid and that surgery won't help me. Is this true?

People with dark, pigmented skin are prone to forming keloids. A keloid is an overgrowth of scar tissue. Keloids, if present in an individual, tend to recur when removed. There is no guarantee that if the present scar is excised you will not form another keloid scar in its place. You should discuss this with your surgeon, and you should know that there *are* options open to you! It may be helpful to have preoperative or postoperative cortisone treatment. In many instances, these measures prevent or at least minimize the formation of keloids. Medical treatment alone or in combination with surgery may be of help. Medical treatment may be especially important when there are symptoms of itching or burning.

I have an ugly, curved, reddish scar on my forehead. Can it be completely removed?

Any incision into skin, whether made by an injury or by a skilled surgeon's scalpel, leaves scar tissue after it heals. Surgery of any kind *always* leaves a scar, no matter how fine and delicate the incision and no matter how well the healing progresses. This is a biological fact of life. In scar-correction surgery, the surgeon carefully plans the operation, taking into account your skin texture, the location of the scar (whether it is on a part of your face where movement occurs or where there is little movement), the width and depth of the scar tissue to be excised, the type of scar (whether it is straight, curved or jagged) and many other factors. The goal of the operation is to *minimize* the present scar, to make it thinner and less conspicuous and, if possible, to have the scar fall within the natural folds of facial skin. But no matter what the surgeon does, you will be left with some minimal scarring.

I had an auto accident two months ago. I now have a scar on my cheek, which really detracts from my appearance. Should I have it corrected now or should I wait?

There is no need to rush into surgery at this time. Two months is not a long time, and the scar will most likely continue to improve over the next few months. In some cases, a scar may heal so well that no surgery is required. The scar is said to mature over this period of time, reaching its final stage between six months and one year. This mature scar can then be approached for revision if necessary. If you have any doubts or questions, or if the scar becomes redder or thicker, you should consult with a plastic surgeon.

I'm a 21-year-old woman and have a small scar on my chin. It bothers me. I know it's not the biggest deal in the world, but I would like to have the scar removed. Am I being vain?

First, the scar cannot be removed. It can be minimized and made to appear less conspicuous. About vanity—there is nothing vain or overly self-indulgent about wanting to appear your best. Assuming your scar is visible and is an annoyance to you, you should certainly feel free to consult with a plastic surgeon to discuss the realistic chances that your scar can be minimized. Remember, no one, if given the choice, would choose to have a scar or blemish that would detract from his or her appearance.

TWELVE

Looking and Feeling Great

As we stressed earlier in this book, cosmetic facial surgery is only one step in what should be a continuing process—an ongoing program of complete care and well-being. After having taken this important first step, you will want to maintain your improved looks and good feelings. You should think of your cosmetic surgery as the first stage toward a new view of yourself, toward new opportunities and beginnings.

Many plastic surgeons know this and advise postoperative patients to see cosmeticians for advice about improving their makeup. This may include a referral to a hair stylist for a new look to complement or enhance a fine postoperative result. Most cosmetic surgeons work with professionals in these other areas. Your surgeon may suggest that you begin a weight-loss program before cosmetic surgery is seriously considered. He or she may recommend that you consult a nutritionist or an exercise specialist for a program of total self-improvement before or after surgery is performed.

In our view, this is a very sensible approach. After all, why spend time, effort and money to improve the way you look and feel if you are not going to maintain this youthful and vital appearance? The most important thing you can do is to develop the proper mind-set so that you will want to maintain and enhance your new looks and good feelings.

Let's say you had a certain flaw (perhaps the shape of your nose or chin, or a sagging neckline) that you have surgically corrected. After your operation, it will help if you can develop new attitudes about your new look or, really, about your new self.

Perhaps you avoided certain clothing styles. Or maybe you shied away from certain social situations because of concern about your nose or chin. If you develop a renewed sense of yourself, you may be willing to try new things. Take chances on new situations. Try a new hair style or a new type of clothing. Go to that party or begin that long-delayed project. These activities may add new dimensions to your effort to improve both your appearance and your feelings about yourself.

Hopefully, your experience with cosmetic surgery will have increased your awareness of your overall looks, fitness and feelings. Your surgery should be a positive first step on the road to personal growth.

A number of studies have shown that most people with a cosmetic flaw feel better after having had it surgically corrected. They look better than they did before the surgery, and they *feel* better about their looks. As a result they feel better about *themselves*.

The decision to have cosmetic surgery is a major move toward self-improvement. Whatever benefits you derive from this step should be maintained and enhanced so that they have lasting value for you. This means taking on a mind-set which is receptive to new, positive changes in your life. Cosmetic facial surgery should be the first major step to a whole new *you*!

Index

Acne scars, 146
Acupuncture, 121
Adrenaline, 45
After-care, 33
Age spots, 146
Aging
  ear problems and, 158
  eyelids and, 86, 87
  forehead lines and, 129
  rhinoplasty and, 54
  speed of, 116–17
  See also Face-lifts
Allergies, 65, 69
  face-lifts and, 124
  to Zyderm, 150
Alcohol, excessive use of, 38
Altered state of consciousness, fear
  of, 47
American Society of Plastic and Reconstructive Surgeons, 16–17,
  127
Analgesics, 138, 142–43
Anemia, 122
Anesthesia, 33, 44–49
  aftereffects of, 46
  for blepharoplasty, 89–90, 94
  for dermabrasion, 146–47
  for ear surgery, 157–58
  fear of, 33
  frequently asked questions about,
    30, 47–48
  general, 44, 48, 158
  local, 44
  not eating before, 43
  for rhinoplasty, 56–57
Anesthesiologist, 44, 48–49
Animation of face, excessive, 132
Antibiotics, 61, 113

Anticoagulants, 122
Anxiety about surgery, 32–33
  anesthesia and, 44–46, 48
Argon laser, 161
Arteries, hardening of, 38
Arthritis, 150
Aspirin, 29–30, 138, 142
Asthma, 69
Atherosclerosis, 38
Attitudes, patient's, 23–24
Autoimmune diseases, 150

Beauty marks, 141
Bereavement, face-lifts and, 123–24
Blacks, rhinoplasty for, 71–72
Bleeding
  adrenaline to minimize, 45
  after blepharoplasty, 91, 95
  after brow and forehead surgery,
    137
  diseases causing, 122
  after face-lift, 108, 109, 113
  medications promoting, 30
  from nose, after rhinoplasty, 59, 61
Blepharoplasty, 85–100
  anesthesia for, 89–90, 94
  brow surgery and, 129–30, 133,
    136
  complications of, 92, 95–96
  cost of, 92, 94
  face-lifts and, 120
  frequently asked questions about,
    92–100
  postoperative period, 90–91
  reactions to, 92
  surgical procedure for, 88–89
  timing of, 86–87

Blind referrals, 15–16
Blues, post-op, 35–36
    after face-lift, 111–13
Board certification, 16
Breathing problems, 54, 56, 65
Brow and forehead surgery, 129–38
    blepharoplasty and, 129–30, 133, 136
    complications of, 137
    frequently asked questions about, 137–38
    postoperative period, 138
    surgical procedures in, 133–37
Brow wrinkles, 118
Bruising, *see* Discoloration
Burn scars, 160

Cataract surgery, 97
Change, psychology of, 34–35
Cheek augmentation, 77, 80
Chemical peeling, 139–46
    complications of, 144
    for crow's-feet, 125
    for dark coloring beneath eyes, 99
    of ear lobes, 158
    face-lifts and, 119
    fees for, 146
    for forehead lines, 133
    frequently asked questions about, 144–46
    preoperative procedures for, 141
    procedures in, 142
    postoperative period, 143
Childhood ear surgery during, 156–158, 162–64
Chin augmentation
    complications of, 78
    cost of, 83
    lips and, 159
    postoperative period, 78
    rhinoplasty and, 65, 75–77
    surgical procedure in, 77–78
Chin reduction, 79–80, 82, 83
Clinics, 18, 20–21
    blepharoplasty in, 90
    fees of, 33
Clothing styles, 170
Collagen treatments, 140, 149–54
    for forehead lines, 133
    frequently asked questions about, 153–54
    for scar correction, 161

Communication, establishing, 25, 26
Complications
    of blepharoplasty, 92, 95–96
    of brow and forehead surgery, 137
    of cheek augmentation, 80
    of chemical peeling, 144
    of chin augmentation, 78
    of dermabrasion, 147
    of face-lifts, 113–14
    of rhinoplasty, 61–63
Consultations, 17–41
    for blepharoplasty, 87
    for ear surgery, 162
    establishing rapport in, 25
    esthetic assessment in, 26–28
    for face-lift, 104–5
    fees for, 40
    fees and arrangements discussed in, 33–34
    patient attitudes and, 23–24
    preoperative considerations in, 29–31
    questions frequently asked in, 19–22, 38–41
    for rhinoplasty, 54
    timing of surgery and, 30–33
Contact lenses, 98
Corrugator muscles, 131, 133
    weakening of, 136–37
Cortisone treatment, 165
Cosmeticians, 169
Costs, *see* Fees
Counseling, *see* Psychological counseling
Credentials of surgeons, 16
Crow's-feet, 125
Cysts, 92

Depression
    after face-lift, 111–13
    postoperative, 35–36, 39–40
Dermabrasion, 139–40, 146–47
    complications of, 147
    cost of, 148
    face-lifts and, 119
    for forehead lines, 133
    frequently asked questions about, 148
    procedure for, 146–47
    for scar correction, 161
Deviated septum, 65, 66, 72
Diabetes, 122

Diet, 37
    after face-lift, 109
    for preoperative patients, 30
Directory of Medical Specialists, 16
Discoloration
    after blepharoplasty, 91, 95
    after brow and forehead surgery,
        137
    after face-lift, 109, 115
Double chin, 124
Doubts about surgery, 20, 31

Ear, nose and throat specialists, 16
Ear surgery, 155–59
    frequently asked questions about,
        162–65
Ectropion, 92, 95
Esthetic assessment, 26–28, 39
    for rhinoplasty, 54
Exercises, facial, 120–21
Expectations
    about face-lifts, 104, 111
    realistic, 24, 35, 38–39
    unrealistic, 36, 40
Eyebrows, *see* Brow and forehead
        surgery
Eyeglasses after rhinoplasty, 59
Eyelid surgery, *see* Blepharoplasty
Eyelid wrinkles and bags, causes of,
        85–86

Face-lifts, 101–27
    brow and forehead surgery and,
        136
    chemical peeling and, 140, 145,
        146
    choosing surgeon for, 16
    collagen treatments and, 150
    complications of, 113–14
    consultations before, 104–5
    cost of, 115
    depression after, 111–13
    frequently asked questions about,
        115–27
    medical conditions and, 122–23
    myths about, 22
    postoperative period, 108–11
    preoperative procedures in, 106–7
    repeat, 117, 120
    surgical procedure in, 106–8
    timing of, 101–4, 117
    weight control after, 37

Facial contouring, 75–83
    chin, 77–79
    cheeks, 80
    cost of, 83
    frequently asked questions about,
        81–83
    harmony and, 75–76
    photographs for studying, 76–77
Facial nerve, injury to, 113–14
False eyelashes, 99
Family members
    blepharoplasty and, 98
    at consultation, 30, 40–41
    having surgery to please, 23
    reactions of, 34
    rhinoplasty and, 69–71, 73
Family physician
    preoperative examination by, 43,
        106
    surgeons recommended by, 15–16
Fat-sculpting, 106
Fear
    of anesthesia, 47
    of surgery, 21, 32–33
Fees, 17, 18, 33–34
    for blepharoplasty, 92, 94
    for chemical peeling, 146
    for consultations, 40
    for dermabrasion, 148
    for face-lifts, 115
    for facial contouring, 83
    for rhinoplasty, 65–66
Flaws
    insignificant, 69–70
    reality of, 23
Follow-up care, 18, 33
Food and Drug Administration
        (FDA), 81, 149, 150
Forehead lines, collagen treatment
        for, 153
Forehead surgery, *see* Brow and fore-
        head surgery
Friends
    having surgery to please, 23
    reactions of, 34
    surgeons recommended by, 15
Frontalis muscle, 130–32
    weakening of, 136

General anesthesia, 44, 48
    for ear surgery, 158
Glaucoma, 97

Goals, patient's, 24
Guilt
  about face-lift, 123
  about surgery, 20

Hair loss after face-lift, 118
Hair style, 37, 169, 170
Hardening of arteries, 38
Harmony, facial, 75–76
Hay fever, 69
Healing process
  after chemical peeling, 143
  after face-lift, 109
  in facial contouring, 80, 81
  after rhinoplasty, 58–60
Health insurance plans, 18, 33
  blepharoplasty and, 94
  face-lifts and, 116
  rhinoplasty and, 67
Heart disease, 122, 141
Hematoma, 113
High blood pressure, 122
Hospital
  blepharoplasty in, 90, 94
  charges of, 18, 33
  face-lifts in, 108–9, 116, 127
  provisions for cosmetic surgery pa-
    tients in, 20–21
Hyperpigmentation
  after chemical peeling, 144
  after dermabrasion, 147, 148
  of eyelids, 99
Hypnosis, 46, 47
Hypoallergenic makeup, 143

Imperfections, reality of, 23
Infection
  after blepharoplasty, 92
  after brow and forehead surgery,
    137
  after chin augmentation, 78
  after face-lift, 113
  after rhinoplasty, 61
Insurance coverage, *see* Health insurance plans
Intravenous catheter, 43–44, 47
  during face-lift operation, 107
  during rhinoplasty operation, 57
Irregular heart beat, 122, 141
Isometric exercises, 137–38, 153

Jaw reshaping, 78–79

Keloids, 165–66
Kidney disease, 122, 141

Laboratory tests, 29, 43
  before face-lift, 106, 122
Lasers, 161–62
Lethargy, postoperative, 46
Lips, adjustment of, 159–61, 164
Liquid silicone, 149–50, 153–54
Liver disorders, 141
Local anesthesia, 44
  for blepharoplasty, 90, 94
  for ear surgery, 158
Lupus erythematosis, 150

Makeup, 37, 169
  after chemical peeling, 143, 144
  after face-lift, 110
Medications
  informing surgeon about, 29–30
  intravenous catheter for adminis-
    tering, 44, 47, 49
  for postoperative pain, 58
Medical assessment, 26
  for rhinoplasty, 54
Medical-grade photographs, 26
Medical history, 29
  face-lift and, 105, 122
  rhinoplasty and, 54
Medical societies, referrals from, 16
Milia, 92
Mini-lift, 120
Motivation for surgery, 23
  rhinoplasty, 69, 70
Muscles, repositioning of, 106
Myopia, 99–100
Myths about surgery, 22
  rhinoplasty, 59

Nausea, postoperative, 46
Near-sightedness, 99–100
Nerve, facial, 113–14
Nevi, 141
Nose, basic anatomy of, 55–56
Nose job, *see* Rhinoplasty
Nosebleeds, 59, 61, 62
Numbness
  after brow and forehead surgery,
    137
  after face-lift, 114
Nurse-anesthetist, 44, 48
Nutrition, 37

Occlusive dressing, 142
Office setting, 18, 20
    ear lobe repair in, 159
Ophthalmologists, 16
    blepharoplasty by, 96
Otolaryngologists, 16
Otoplasty, 155–59
    frequently asked questions about,
        162–65
Outpatient facilities, 18, 20–21
    blepharoplasty in, 94
    face-lifts in, 109, 116, 127
Over-the-counter medications, 29

Packing, nasal, 57
Para-amino benzoic acid (PABA),
    60, 111, 145
Payment in advance, 18
Personality, changes in, 64
Phenol, 141, 142, 146
Photographs
    examination of, 26–28, 39
    before face-lifts, 105
    for studying facial contours, 76–77
Physical examination, 43
    before chemical peeling, 141
    before face-lift, 106, 122
    of nose, 54
Plastic surgeons, *see* Surgeons
Pores, enlarged, 141
Port wine stains, 161
Postoperative period
    aftereffects of anesthesia in, 46
    after blepharoplasty, 90–91
    after brow and forehead surgery,
        138
    after cheek augmentation, 80
    after chemical peeling, 143
    after chin augmentation, 78
    depression during, 35–36
    explanation of, 17, 29, 30, 33–34
    after face-lift, 108–11, 127
    after rhinoplasty, 57–60
Preoperative photographs, 26–29, 39
Preoperative procedures, 43–44
    for chemical peeling, 141
    explanation of, 29
    for face-lift, 106–7
    for rhinoplasty, 57
Protruding ears, 155–59
Psychological counseling, 32–33
    before blepharoplasty, 87–88

before ear surgery, 157
face-lifts and, 103–4, 111
for postoperative depression, 35–
    36
Pug noses, 72

Rapport, establishing, 25
Realistic expectations, 24, 25, 38–39
Reconstructive surgeons, *see* Sur-
    geons
Recovery period
    presence of family members dur-
        ing, 30
    See also Postoperative period
Referrals, 15–16
Rhinoplasty, 53–73
    anesthesia for, 56–57
    anxiety about, 32–33
    chin augmentation and, 65, 75–77
    complications of, 61–63
    consultation for, 54
    cost of, 65–66
    depression after, 35
    esthetic assessment before, 26–29
    frequently asked questions about,
        63–73
    motivation for, 23
    myths about, 22
    postoperative period, 57–60
    preoperative procedure for, 57
    surgical procedure in, 54–56
    timing of, 53–54, 67–68
    unsatisfactory results of, 63, 67

Sagging, causes of, 101
Scar correction, 160–61
    frequently asked questions about,
        165–67
Scarring
    after blepharoplasty, 89, 91, 92, 95
    after chemical peeling, 144, 145
    after dermabrasion, 144
    after ear surgery, 158, 165
    after face-lift, 113, 114, 118–19
    after rhinoplasty, 67
Scowling, 130–32
Sedation, 44–47
    during blepharoplasty, 90
    during face-lift operation, 107
    during rhinoplasty, 57

Self-alienation after rhinoplasty, 73
Self-esteem
　face-lifts and, 104
　rhinoplasty and, 61, 64
Septum
　deviated, 65, 66, 72
　reduction in height of, 56
Shaving after face-lift, 122
Silicone, liquid, 149–50, 153–54
Silicone implants
　for cheek augmentation, 80
　for chin augmentation, 77–78
　migration of, 81
Skin thickness
　chemical peeling and, 141
　face-lifts and, 105, 119, 121–22
　rhinoplasty and, 55
Skin slough, 113
Smell, sense of, 63
Smoking, 38
Sneezing after rhinoplasty, 59
Specialists, 16
Splint, nasal, 57, 58, 72
　removal of, 60, 61
Spouse, *see* Family members
Squinting
　crow's-feet and, 125
　scowl lines and, 125
Steroids, 122, 143
Sun exposure, 38
　after blepharoplasty, 97
　after chemical peeling, 143
　after dermabrasion, 144
　after face-lift, 110–11, 118, 124
　after rhinoplasty, 59–60
Surgeons
　consultations with, *see* Consultations
　credentials of, 16, 127
　referrals to, 15–16
　training and qualifications of, 16–17
Surgical procedures
　for blepharoplasty, 88–89
　for brow and forehead, 133–37
　for cheek augmentation, 80
　for chemical peeling, 142–43
　for chin augmentation, 77–78
　for dermabrasion, 146–47
　for ears, 155–59
　explanation of, 17, 29, 30
　for face-lifts, 106–8

　for lip adjustments, 159–61
　for rhinoplasty, 54–56
　for scar correction, 160–61
Swelling, postoperative, 34
　after blepharoplasty, 90–92
　after chemical peeling, 142–43, 146
　after chin augmentation, 78
　after chin reduction, 82
　diet to reduce, 30
　after face-lift, 108, 109, 113, 115, 125
　after rhinoplasty, 57–60, 63, 66

Tattoos, laser treatment of, 162
Tests, *see* Laboratory tests
Timing of surgery, 30–33
　blepharoplasty, 86–87, 95
　face-lifts, 101–4, 117
　rhinoplasty, 53–54, 67–68
Titanium dioxide, 60, 111, 145
Topical anesthesia, 147
Tranquilizers
　preoperative, 44
　during surgery, 47
　See also Sedation
Twilight sleep, 45
　for blepharoplasty, 90
Tylenol, 142

Valium, 44
Vision, blurring of, after blepharoplasty, 91, 92
Vitamin E, 29–30
Vomiting, postoperative, 46

Weight control, 37, 169
　face-lifts and, 119
Wisdom teeth, removal of, 82–83
Wrinkles
　brow, 118
　causes of, 101
　on ear lobes, 158
　removal of, *see* Chemical peeling; Dermabrasion
　skin thickness and, 121–22

X-rays, 43
　before chin reduction, 78

Zinc oxide, 60, 111, 145
Zyderm, 150–52